"Humanistic care is the result of a colla [...] including clinical chaplains. Gordon Hil [...] case and provides a practical framework for chaplains to document the state of the patient's human spirit in the face of uncertainty and adversity in the medical chart. This act of 'humanizing' the medical chart creates the climate for spiritual care to complement medical care and therefore promote healing. This book is a must-read for every member of the interdisciplinary medical team."

—*Juan C. Iregui, MD Palliative Medicine & Ethics*

"Magnificent work—a must-read for healthcare professionals. Hilsman's artful analysis of spirituality fills a gap in the caring professions' knowledge base. Providing insight into healing, Hilsman's theory draws the reader into recognizing what makes up the human spirit from surprising angles."

—*Brenda Miller, MSN, RN, BC-NE, Nursing Director,*
Massachusetts General Hospital, Boston, Massachusetts

"Weaving together a lifetime of experience with a growing body of research, Gordon Hilsman has crafted a guide that proves beneficial to both the novice clinical pastoral education student as well as the seasoned clinical spiritual care giver. This book, both expansive in breadth and thoughtful in depth, is warmly accessible yet never trite, making it also a significant resource for interdisciplinary teams interested in the practice of spiritual care."

—*Trace Haythorn, PhD, MDiv, Executive Director,*
The Association for Clinical Pastoral Education Inc.

"Kudos for *Spiritual Care in Common Terms*, an inspiring and self-revealing look at the science and art of spiritual care. Hilsman reveals the best-kept secrets of professional chaplaincy and openly welcomes all who care for the body, mind, and spirit of the human person. A must-read!"

—*Tim Serban, Chief Mission Integration Officer at Providence Health*
& Services, Oregon, National Volunteer Lead at American Red Cross
Disaster Spiritual Care, author, and Board-Certified Chaplain

"I have had the privilege over recent years in diverse professional learning settings to experience Gordon examining this topic of capturing in common language the soul of another so that this vital knowledge can be understood by the multidisciplinary care team to inform goals and plans of care. Combining theory, cases, numerous examples of goals of care, and spiritual care wisdom honed from years of clinical education and practice, Gordon masterfully provides (using his criteria for quality chart notes) a very understandable, significantly substantive, and exceptionally readable volume that will serve very well the chaplains and health care professionals to whom he has devoted his life for the benefit of the care recipient's healing and wholeness."

—*David A. Lichter, D.Min., Executive Director, NACC*

"This is a marvelous and important book. In lucid prose, Gordon Hilsman explains the importance of succinct, earthy spiritual assessment notes for the medical record. He shows us the how and the why, and reminds us how important it is to create an image in the chart of the entirety of a person. The patients we all serve, and our poor beleaguered healthcare system, will be the better for listening to his call, recounted with warmth, wisdom, empathy, and good humor."

—*David K. Urion, M.D., FAAN, Director of Education and Residency Training Programs in Child Neurology and Neurodevelopmental Disabilities, Co-Chair, Ethics Advisory Committee, Boston Children's Hospital*

"Spirituality of patients is an essential domain of whole-person care. Patients often suffer in silence; that suffering or spiritual distress must be recognized and treated. Professional chaplains are essential members of the healthcare team. It is critical that they communicate verbally and in the chart note the spiritual needs of the patient, how they are addressing that need and what outcomes the team should look for to help the patient heal. Spiritual Care in Common Terms offers the language and format for chaplains to communicate this clinical aspect of spiritual care that can be understood in the reductionist clinical framework but keeps the patient's inner narrative in the forefront of their care for all members to provide compassionate care for our patients. This is a must-read for not only chaplains but for other members of the interdisciplinary team."

—*Christina Puchalski, MD, FACP, FAAHPM*

SPIRITUAL CARE
in Common Terms

of related interest

**Assessing and Communicating the Spiritual
Needs of Children in Hospital**
A new guide for healthcare professionals and chaplains
Alister Bull
ISBN 978 1 84905 637 3
eISBN 978 1 78450 116 7

Critical Care
Delivering Spiritual Care in Healthcare Contexts
Edited by Jonathan Pye, Peter Sedgwick and Andrew Todd
ISBN 978 1 84905 497 3
eISBN 978 0 85700 901 2

Spiritual Care in Practice
Case Studies in Healthcare Chaplaincy
Edited by George Fitchett and Steve Nolan
ISBN 978 1 84905 976 3
eISBN 978 0 85700 876 3

Spiritual Care with Sick Children and Young People
**A handbook for chaplains, paediatric health
professionals, arts therapists and youth workers**
Paul Nash, Kathryn Darby and Sally Nash
ISBN 978 1 84905 389 1
eISBN 978 1 78450 063 4

Spiritual Care at the End of Life
The Chaplain as a 'Hopeful Presence'
Steve Nolan
ISBN 978 1 84905 199 6
ISBN 978 0 85700 513 7

SPIRITUAL CARE

in Common Terms

How Chaplains Can Effectively
Describe the Spiritual Needs of Patients
in Medical Records

Gordon J. Hilsman, D.Min.

Foreword by James H. Gunn

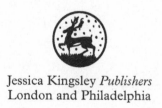

Jessica Kingsley *Publishers*
London and Philadelphia

First published in 2017
by Jessica Kingsley Publishers
73 Collier Street
London N1 9BE, UK
and
400 Market Street, Suite 400
Philadelphia, PA 19106, USA

www.jkp.com

Library of Congress Cataloging in Publication Data
A CIP catalog record for this book is available from the Library of Congress

British Library Cataloguing in Publication Data
A CIP catalogue record for this book is available from the British Library

ISBN 978 1 78592 724 9
eISBN 978 1 78450 369 7

Printed and bound in the United States

To Lincoln Ure, colleague, consultant, consultor, and glorious friend

Contents

Foreword

Spiritual care departments have come a long way in the past 50 years, and yet, not so far when it comes to establishing a culture that provides a coherent, dependable and understandable way of charting the work of chaplains and spiritual care providers. Gordon Hilsman, in *Spiritual Care in Common Terms*, argues for a coherent practice of writing a chart note for the healthcare interdisciplinary team (IDT). His call to write a foreword for his book came to me out of the blue in the midst of a satisfying retirement. The reading of his text has transported me back over the last 50 years of my ministry and a review of clinical pastoral education and much of the literature in the field of pastoral/spiritual care.

How should a chaplain document her pastoral care contacts in a multidisciplinary healthcare setting? It wasn't so long ago that chaplains were forbidden to access the medical chart, let alone enter a record of a visit. And then, "in the beginning" there were separate pages in some departments or ancillary pages in others for chaplains, later known as spiritual care. In my residency program the pink pages were included in the inpatient chart but were removed from the chart when it was sent to medical records for filing. The pink sheets were returned to the chaplain's office where they were used, or not, for supervision of intern and resident chaplains.

It was 50 years ago (spring 1966) that I took my first unit of clinical pastoral education in a juvenile detention facility in Chicago. It was the end of my second year of seminary; my professor of pastoral care was Carroll Wise. His book *The Meaning of Pastoral Care* helped shape my approach and understanding of my ministry. Providing care to persons at "the point of their need" became the standard by which I measured my pastoral practice. Articulating my ministry, interventions, and the outcomes of the care has been a lifelong process of learning. Sharing descriptions of my work with an IDT has been the object of many hours of individual and group supervision. The impetus for writing coherent chart notes developed with increased acceptance and integration of spiritual care in the healthcare environment.

At the end of my career, I phased into retirement in several stages. I gave away portions of my professional library to two different clinical pastoral education (CPE) libraries and the remainder to students or some local "used" book stores. Our decision to live "full time" in a motor home did not fit well into my obsessive need to collect books. I am still an inveterate reader, but my reading now tends to be borrowed library books loaned to my e-reader and then returned. Public libraries do not have a substantial collection of books on pastoral/spiritual care, so I have been engrossed with the likes of Lee Childs' Jack Reacher, and his ilk.

After Hilsman's call, I was intrigued and pleased that I could read the draft of his book on my computer, and pleased to be reading again literature growing out of a career that provided intellectual stimulation and personal satisfaction and enrichment. What a change from the days of my residency when copies of verbatim reports were churned out still wet on a spirit duplicator machine! (If the reader does not know what that is, talk to an "old" teacher before they are all gone, although information about them is available via Google.) As a result of reading Hilsman's work I have been transported back through the decades of my career and the various seasons and themes of said career in terms of interests, fads, and passions. Essentially, I have relived the pastoral care literature and movement from the 1960s, 1970s, 1980s, 1990s, and the first decade of the current century. This reliving has all been in my mind and my soul, since I no longer have access to the books that have been so formative and informative. I am pleasantly surprised that Google can find names and publication dates and resources for reordering these if I so choose!

Tomorrow or next week I will remember another author who should have been mentioned here, but for now the following persons and resources have made their impact on my developing understanding and practice. Of course, the pastoral care fathers of Wise, Clinebell, Oates, Madden, and others were the "required" reading of the early days. Clebsch and Jaekle published *Pastoral Care in Historical Perspective* in the mid-1960s, providing a framework for understanding our work centered on the themes of *healing, sustaining, guiding,* and *reconciling.* These themes have been substantial and lasting in that they have undergirded the movement for the past 50 years as they did in the "historical perspective." Some have suggested that we should add *transforming* to that list. Maybe there are others?

Admittedly, one major emphasis of the movement grew out of a psychodynamic understanding of human personality. In the mid-1970s, Paul Pruyser, a clinical psychologist and a Presbyterian layperson who was intimately involved with the CPE program in Topeka, Kansas, published his book *The Minister as Diagnostician.* My memory of his motive for writing this book was that he rather despaired over clergy who tried to sound like psychoanalytic clinicians and chose to write this book encouraging clergy to use the language of faith rather than psychology. His work served as an important corrective for the movement in pushing the pastoral practitioner toward listening for the human narrative in terms of their engagement of the faith journey in the broad sweep of theological themes.

In the 1980s, Elisabeth McSherry, M.D. began her work with chaplains around the issue of spiritual assessment. Her work, along with that of Greg Stoddard, George Fitchett, Gary Berg, and many others thrust the movement into a new phase of development in which assessment was done along a consistent frame of reference that identified a person's relationship to the holy, whether or not the person had a sense of community, whether or not the person had a sense of hopefulness, and whether or not the person had a sense of spiritual pain.

Pastoral care researchers Fitchett, VandeCreek, Handzo, Gleason, and many others began to collect data about assessment, interventions, and outcomes. Physicians became interested in the medical outcomes observed in patients who came from faith-based backgrounds and practice. Benson, Matthews, Dossey, Koenig, and Puchalski were prodigious writers and speakers on the pastoral care circuit as they were active in the medical community. The *Journal of Health Care Chaplaincy* continues to make important contributions to the field.

Chaplains have known their work is significant and life changing for patients and their families. They have not always had the courage to speak to their convictions in language common to, and with the kind of evidence demanded in, a scientific environment. Sometimes they have remained silent when their observations and knowledge of a patient/family dynamic would have been helpful to the IDT. Sometimes they have offered meaningless tidbits of family gossip that did not aid the clinician's understanding of a patient's need.

And now, Hilsman's work is designed to sharpen the dialog with members of the IDT via a carefully crafted chart note that communicates the essence of the spiritual care encounter in humanistic terms that will likely be read by members of the IDT *and* contribute to the care of the patient in the hospital or clinic. Chapter 1 asks and answers the question of "why" record the "intangible" in a healthcare culture that is fixated on those things that can be known and measured.

Chapter 2 spells out the "theory" for this work based on an understanding of humanism in four universal sources (Interpersonal, Personal, Transcendent, and Communal Spirituality) of personal narratives.

Chapter 3 identifies the "content" of the chart note based on 22 spiritual needs common to hospitalized persons. These 22 needs are arrayed in four groups identified as: emotional support needs; major loss needs; religious and spiritual practice needs; and referral needs.

Chapter 4 suggests a "format" for the chart note that captures the "soul" of the person in an "elegant" sentence that gets to the heart of the patient's narrative as it relates to the issues and concerns surrounding this healthcare crisis.

Chapter 5 describes the process involved in "extracting the relevant" factors in creating the note by considering the readers of the note and provides considerations for constructing the note. Chapter 6 focuses on "outcomes" from a phenomenological point of view. Hilsman reports on some departmental studies that support and reinforce his theory and suggests that more rigorous and robust studies be done.

The Epilogue summarizes this body of work in terms of the skill set needed for becoming a competent spiritual care practitioner. Hilsman's focus on the ways his theories have evolved from care provided in addiction and palliative care programs is a core component in understanding and implementing his suggestions for crafting a humanistic note for the IDT.

As history bears out, these will not be the last words on this subject but they are an important contribution to the spiritual care movement and the importance of getting the human narrative back into the practice of medicine. This book will be of significant help to students and serious practitioners. It will be of particular help for those who work with patients over a longer period of time than the "average" hospital patient. It will be of help to practitioners who have intense and meaningful encounters in the clinic or hospital. For practitioners who are not currently writing notes or communicating with the IDT this book may be an inspiration to change their practice.

Thus Hilsman's emphasis on the "humanistic" rather than "religious" interpretation and recording one's assessment and interventions is the next necessary move in the ever-changing role of the spiritual care provider in a medical IDT. At the same time, the sharing of his own personal narrative and several examples of colleagues and patients give ample evidence of the importance of reporting and recording specific religious practices when reporting an encounter to the IDT, especially when such practices convey the essence of the human spirit or soul of a specific individual.

If the reader is looking for a recipe for crafting a chart note for the medical record, she will be disappointed. If the reader is looking to be challenged to deeper thought and a wrestling with the complex issues of integrating her spiritual conversation into a conceptual narrative that will honestly portray the art of one's hearing into a brief note that will actually be read by busy clinicians, she will be rewarded with new work and the need to stay in a learning community (e.g. Hemenway 1996) that will continue to push this discipline into the future where integrative medicine will involve and care for the whole person.

James H. Gunn, Association for Clinical Pastoral Education (ACPE) Supervisor, Retired

Acknowledgments

There have been four kinds of relationships that have contributed to the process of writing this book—mentors, encouragers, consultors, and supporters. I am so grateful to all of these and to others who were not as central to this project but did assist me along the way.

Key mentors arrived when this student was ready. Bernie Pennington and Bob Jais dedicated considerable time and concerted effort to help me learn clinical supervision and build its identity into my bones. Social worker Joan Armstrong, who like Bernie and Bob had completed considerable psychoanalysis, gave me confidence from her supervisory perspective from outside pastoral care as a clinical social worker. Some years before, Orwoll (Oz) Anderson inspired me towards clinical ministry in my first introduction to clinical pastoral education with a highly humanistic approach to helping people that emphasized direct observation, accurate description, and immediate processing of relationship events. Jim Anderson modeled the human-to-human relationship for me so well, before he died at 51. I was so fortunate to have found them all at the right time of my life.

A few people sprang up to encourage me at moments that seemed ordinary at the time, but in retrospect lifted me up and forward as a spiritual care practitioner and as a writer. CEO Lowell Miller saw potential in me and hired me as a chaplain, as I had exited from the active Catholic priesthood, after two years of mostly being lost. Mary Jane O'Neil and Stephanie Wohrle helped me understand the path of addicts to recovery and its maintenance, as well as grasp the art of confrontation. Noel Brown's comment that I was one of the few clear thinkers in the field of clinical ministry, and Rock Stack's remark that I really know how to write a paragraph, were quietly instrumental in my beginning to write in my 50s. Herbert Anderson was the first to invite me to write an article, that one for the *Dictionary of Pastoral Care* on laicization, a topic he correctly discerned would fit my situation at the time. As these moments now emerge from the fog of lagging memory I multiply my appreciation for them.

Palliative care physician Juan Iregui connected with me in uncommon ways over scores of walks above Chambers Bay golf course, picking one another's brains about people as patients, concepts for relationships, and outrageous boyish humor, privately making fun of one another and anybody we pleased. In his 30s and 40s he boosted my spirit and prodded this publication during my 60s with an unexplainably perspicacious grasp of who I am. Epidemiologist and CEO Rick MacCornack did something similar over breakfast and lunch. Friendship indeed does feed the soul like nothing else.

Consultation on this book has truly brought shape to it, particularly from palliative care pediatrician Pat O'Malley at Massachusetts General, clinical pastoral education (CPE) supervisor Sandy Walker in Portland, Oregon, and Glori Schneider, a former student and sharp critic of writing, spiritual care, and its management. I am grateful to Garrett Starmer for the hospital chaplaincy data that forms the illustrative content of Chapter 6; to Patricia McElroy whose combined experience as an attorney and a chaplain educator helped with Chapter 5; and to Bonnie

Pat McDougal Olson in New York for her feedback on the book's later stages. Nurses Ashley Richter, Brady Hilsman, and Nancy, my wife, made significant validating and critical comments that contributed heavily to the intricacies of this book. Hospital system spiritual care leaders Jennifer Paquette, Becca Parkins, Terry Hollister, and NACC executive director David Lichter have been most encouraging and helpful with networking opportunities in presenting this material.

Consultation on my thinking about this specific topic over the years has come largely from four colleagues who have validated and challenged my work and theirs, in a biannual peer group meeting at our house in Fircrest for many years. That practice has been the lifeblood of my continued creativity, particularly as this book project has progressed—Sandy Walker, Lisa Nordlander, Wes McIntyre and my best friend of 20 years Lincoln Ure, God rest his soul. I still stand together with them in this consultative group with confirming support and prodding confrontation flowing freely. I treasure them and that part of my life.

Such consultation would be much more difficult and costly without my wife Nancy's support and hospitality at our house. She has also put up with my intellectualizing and my writing mind so often when emotional connection would have been by far her preference. Thank God for her and 37 years of the crucible of loving and contending that makes up a vigorous love life. May I truly retire soon.

Preface

This book is an effort to foster greater integration of spiritual perspectives into healthcare culture. It is founded on the belief that what happens inside people when they are hospitalized has a significant effect on their healing from what brought them there and often stimulates positive changes in the rest of their lives. The current practice of surveying patients by phone after discharge ignores the opportunity to promote healing while hospitalized and never catches and responds helpfully to the actual "patient experience." Spiritual care can do that and often does, despite the sparsity of chaplaincy in US hospitals.

Spiritual Care in Common Terms began as an effort to help chaplains and pastoral care students better represent their spiritual care of people in the medical record. In the writing it became more than that. It made room for clinicians to begin writing spiritual care notes of their own. I met Pat O'Malley, a palliative care pediatrician who works in the emergency department of Massachusetts General Hospital. She was writing her chart notes with an obvious spiritual care bent. She had completed one unit of clinical pastoral education, it appealed to her, and she adapted what she learned there to her charting. When an electronic medical record was initiated at that world-class hospital, she heard interdisciplinary team colleagues worried that she might change her style of charting for the sake of uniformity. They liked her human-to-human tone and description of patient issues about medical challenges, troubling relationships, and ultimate values.

Let me be clear about for whom this book is intended, lest its presentation confuse you. Its target audience is anyone who sometimes thinks that thoughts about transcendence, persistent worries, and interpersonal issues have a serious effect on the healing of people. It is for physicians who find that folks come to them when their human spirit is alarmed enough by a physical concern that they seek help to find out why, but often can't optimally use that help because of elusive, complex behavioral problems. It is for nurses who so commonly work with patients who seem to sabotage their own health that they get frustrated but keep on working on their mound of cases quietly mystified by the ways that the inner world of people affects their health. It is for chaplains who work in relative isolation among clinicians because they so poorly communicate in common terms what they do for patients. And it is for medical social workers who have their own language in which to help people negotiate systems of assistance while wondering about why religion seems so solid in some people's lives and yet so dysfunctional in its intended role of augmenting their human spirits.

The notion of spiritual care in common terms has been brewing in my mind all my life, although only consciously so for the past three decades. As a quiet, mostly well-behaved and markedly inward boy, I found the virtues of Catholic culture fascinating, mostly as evident in the lives of biblical characters and saints. My introverted pondering was persistently wondering, "How do you really get those virtues anyhow?" and "Who around me has specific ones, really?" Such thoughts were far from being discussed, or even expressed at the time. But they brewed and simmered beneath and found plenty of processing in preparation for the Catholic priesthood.

As a chemistry major and physics minor I came in touch with the visionary thinking of Teilhard de Chardin and am compelled by it to this day. Here was a scientist, a Jesuit priest, a paleontologist, an enormously creative thinker, who used his science to fashion an evolutionary view of the universe that makes actual big-picture sense. There is no science–religion barrier. There is only one world, with different approaches and varying perspectives to understanding and improving it. Science pecks away glacially at revealing tiny bits of reality and feeding technologists who improve world living conditions. Religion, imperfect and dysfunctional as it is at this point in evolution, at its best uses mystery, teaching, and inspiration to better the human race in a massive evolutionary process moving towards global community and beyond. "Don't be intimidated by esoteric jargon of any of that," I learned. "Decide what you have within you to further this glorious process and get busy at contributing to evolution in your own best way."

It was in an all-male CPE group in Eau Claire, Wisconsin, that I recognized evolution in the immediate moment, a small group collaborating and challenging for the truth about how we actually see one another, and what really happens emotionally between us, and the subjects of our ministry laid bare. Where do you find words to describe people accurately, authentically, and usefully, face to face and in writing? There were no chaplain chart notes then, in the 1970s, but the skills of finding common terms, as well as new concepts that fit so well, were budding in preparation for this book.

But it was in Chicago that I was slammed into the most intense crucible of real, here and now, life-saving spiritual dynamics, in Alcoholics Anonymous (AA) groups all around the city. E.B. was a young African American with an obviously deformed arm and an indomitable spirit that took me to AA meetings to help me learn. It was unethical. The only requirement for attending an actual meeting is an honest desire to stop drinking. I didn't have that, and he knew it. But he liked me and knew that the sacredness of that starkly honest atmosphere was such a gift he couldn't deny it to me as I learned about addiction in the treatment program at Rush St. Luke's Presbyterian Medical Center in which he was the AA coordinator. As a counseling resident in the treatment program I was charged with charting on patients' progress, or lack of it, day to day. Theological terms were useless. Delivering half-hour lectures on spiritual topics to people desperate for radical life change needed common terms. I was gradually finding them. It would be years before I spent over a decade during the 1980s in a treatment program based rigorously on the Twelve Steps of Alcoholics Anonymous. But Chicago was a soul grabbing start.

In the treatment program in Ashland, Wisconsin, based on the Minnesota Model of using the Twelve Steps rigorously, I engaged people about their gut level spirituality as a pivotal part of their recovery. Here we had bi-weekly group sessions of people who needed spiritual perspectives and challenges for their very survival. Most of them had some religious heritage, yet all of them were completely defeated by a simple chemical substance, ethanol, the only one of a class of chemicals that isn't quickly fatal when consumed. If you happen to be one of the 10 percent of people who ought not drink it, it steals everything from your life first before you die of its ravaging effects. Alcoholics were, I was finding out, marvelous people, all of them. Only a few fortunate ones were heroically recovering from a deadly disease that required a deeply spiritual process of change in order to live normal lives.

This book is the current state of my ongoing process of finding common terms for spiritual care. The first chapter asks the question of why one would chart spiritual perspectives in the medical record, which is designed for practical communication of medical and nursing clinicians. It answers that question in six different ways, highlighting the humanistic nature of spiritual care and its essential place in healthcare culture. It offers a conceptual meaning of the term "spiritual" that encompasses all of life, from opening up spiritual care conversations to focusing on the current state of the human spirit, the most useful content of spiritual care chart notes.

Chapter 2 illustrates three dozen universal sources of patient stories that alert a spiritual caregiver who listens personally, not only diagnostically, to the depth of patients' inner experience, positive or negative, bubbling up in a context in which they feel well heard.

There are several spiritual needs that present themselves over and over in hospitalized people. Decades of chaplain experience have shown us that. Chapter 3 presents 22 of them, along with suggested goals of care for each. That framework organizes the immense complexity of spiritual care needs and the advantages of focusing on patient needs rather than chaplain functions or assessment concepts. It suggests descriptive narrative to augment or replace the boxes to check and lines to fill featured in electronic medical records that have been so carefully and diversely fashioned for research and administrative oversight rather than for patient care.

A format for spiritual care chart notes that parallels one used by many physicians is the subject of Chapter 4. A first sentence of every note that intentionally tries to compel the attention of clinicians as substantive and useful begins every note, whether from a first visit with an emergency patient or the tenth with a chronically ill one. "Capturing the soul" of all patients who can converse is the goal of writing chart notes all day long.

The multitude of professional disciplines with some interest in chart notes are the content of Chapter 5, along with some suggestions about the process of writing a chart note narrative. Examples of chart notes are used in Chapters 3, 4, and 5, composites pasted together from actual student and chaplain notes in several healthcare facilities. Nobody should be able to recognize who wrote them about whom.

The final chapter considers the partially observable outcomes of spiritual care conversations. The phenomenological method and humanistic perspectives used throughout the book lead to a way of evaluating spiritual care conversations and the chart notes that result from them. No credible research has been done on the perspectives of this book, and Chapter 6 shows how that research is possible and could be useful to the field of clinical ministry.

The Epilogue attempts to elucidate skills and virtues that need to be developed in anyone purporting to become and remain a spiritual clinician. The competencies for certification by the major US associations of chaplains have served the field well. Yet there remain fully certified chaplains who struggle to work in palliative care, addictions, and hospice programs and actually fail to do so with any significant contributions to the facility missions there. What are the missing skills and essential characteristics that can be learned in formative education and on the job? And how can those be acquired? This book assumes in the reader some mastery of skills of establishing intimate professional rapport with people in personal pain. It focuses more directly on how to represent that care in interdisciplinary writing.

The reader will note that the term "spiritual caregiver" can refer to more than chaplains. There is no firm protectiveness of turf here. There are medical and nursing clinicians who possess a natural aptitude for establishing spiritual conversational rapport and learning to write spiritual care notes, some even including religious issues. They, too, however, need an educational forum for looking closely with stark feedback on their relational proclivities, communication habits, and interpersonal blind spots to largely free them from the prisons of their projections, rationalizations, and intellectualized safe spots. Clinical pastoral education remains the primary and best method for achieving that.

1

Why Record the Intangible in Healthcare Culture?

Humanism, in all its simplicity, is the only genuine spirituality.

ALBERT SCHWEITZER[1]

You're a professional caregiver interested in the spiritual aspect of human care—perhaps a chaplain, or a nurse fascinated with the effect of people's spirituality on their health, or a physician curious about a patient's sharp attitude. You've just finished a substantive conversation with a hospital patient and are headed for the computer program to record salient aspects about it. Wait! Why? What is your best understanding of your motivation to write in the medical record about the elusive, subjective, and intangible aspects of patients' experiences? Even prior to that, how do you understand your own motivation for engaging people personally in the midst of their life difficulties

---

1   Dr. Schweitzer used this assertion in a lecture delivered in French in the Auditorium of Oslo University in 1951 as he accepted the Nobel Peace Prize, first published in *Les Prix Nobel* in 1954 in Stockholm, Sweden.

and investing considerable energy in doing so as a component of a professional career? If those questions have not found solid answers in your formative education or subsequent self-reflection, then now is the time to work them out before further engaging a process to improve what you write about patients in medical charts.

Communication in hospital culture tends to be focused, earthy, and stark. The entire unique milieu of health care persists as highly pragmatic, humanistic, and decisive. In other words: 1) interdisciplinary team (IDT) members tend to focus doggedly on what works rather than what may be ultimately true; 2) they care for any human being who presents herself in medical need; and 3) they make dozens if not hundreds of decisions every day quickly, carefully, and effectively. Anyone purporting to be helping people religiously or spiritually in that culture will need to honor that milieu, embrace it, and learn to engage it on a human-to-human, here-and-now, concrete, and easily understandable level. That person will need to know her role and value it as making a contribution to humanity. And it is becoming increasingly clear that they will need common terms in which to do so.

A major characteristic of spiritual caregivers who work in that culture is a conviction that collaborating with IDT members has solid value. Much of the communicating with IDT members takes place informally, face to face, with one person or a few at a time. But to communicate with all of the IDT members it is necessary to clearly represent spiritual perspectives on patients in the medical record.

But do spiritual points of view even belong in patients' charts? Why should spiritual perspectives become a part of the official medical record at all? There are several excellent answers to that central question.

Spiritual perspectives in the healing process

A management development program being used by a medium-sized healthcare system asked employees several pointed questions in order to give feedback to department directors on their leadership. One of the questions to staff members was, "Do you believe that your work contributes to the mission of this healthcare system?" The spiritual care director was more than appalled when several of the questionnaires from her chaplains answered the question flatly, "No." They did not see their care of patients' inner world, ultimate concerns, and challenges to their very core making a contribution to their healing. "Why is this hospital paying you then?" she asked the entire staff. A great teaching moment had erupted. If spiritual care does help patients heal then its caregivers' notes belong in the charts. If not, then why are they working there?

Spiritual perspectives help patients because they attend to the inner world of people suffering physical challenges. All communication about patients' physical states and treatment processes reveals only a shadow of what is actually happening inside those patients. The emphasis of the entire medical record is, by necessity and by tradition, highly focused on the body. Much of what is happening to a patient's *mind* in understanding, *heart* in emotional experience, and *human spirit* in facing ultimate concerns, simmers beneath. But when a crucial *health event* emerges there almost always arises an accompanying *personal* emergency (from the Latin *emergere* meaning "to rise out or up"). Clinicians have learned in their initial formation to deftly keep patients' feelings and attitudes from influencing their practices too much. Intricate and prolonged interpersonal communication is mostly a distraction to traditional medical and even nursing care.

Hospitals are places, however, that precipitate patients' recognition of and reflection on ultimate concerns. The term healing had almost disappeared from medical journals until palliative care revived it later in the 20th century. Cure rather than care had become physicians' focus as medicine had taken on a more scientific identity. The term "healing" is now more commonly used in a holistic sense with a more psychological nuance, as "a process in the service of the evolution of the whole personality towards ever greater and more complex wholeness" (Egnew 2005). The pragmatic definition we use in this book is *an improvement in an individual's capacity to meet the inherent painful realities of an uncontrollable world with personal resilience, a positive attitude, and realistic expectations of an enjoyable future.* As hospice and palliative care services have vividly discovered, there can be a great deal of healing even where there will be no cure.

The abrupt, temporary vulnerability of hospitalization variously brings to the surface of consciousness the hurts of patients' pasts that have been waiting, mostly unconsciously, for healing. Such healing of past hurts and issues involves verbally processing by telling stories of regrets, resentments, failures, and major losses to carefully listening ears. What new medical specialties—notably hospice, palliative care, and addiction recovery—are discovering is that healing is personal and interpersonal as much as it is physical (Cassell 2012).[2] Healing happens primarily inside a person through engagement from unique relationships touching from the outside.

Spiritual care—with its unique brand of personal rather than diagnostic listening, creative conveyance of empathy, broad-ranging acceptance, non-anxious presence, and studied frameworks of understanding the human spirit—has the potential to enhance the human healing of most people who can still talk and some who no longer can. Somewhere in all significant healing processes is at least one person who has a more than slight appreciation of what it is like for that patient on that day. It may come from a family member, a particularly attuned nurse or a chaplain who listens with genuine interest and a lingering presence to the spoken experience of that patient. Healing processes are not insular. They include a verbal processing element that can change an entire life.

Understanding this can be facilitated by seeing the healing process itself as always including several elements, none of which is totally effective alone. A serious healing event is essentially an uneven confluence

---

2   Cassell has been most vocal in helping improve physicians' and other health professionals' understanding of the human-to-human elements in the process of healing. He cites other pioneers in this endeavor writing in the past 50 years for the transformation of the practice of medicine, including: Michael Balint (1968) *The Doctor, His Patient and the Illness.* London: Pitman Medical Publishing; George L. Engel (1977) 'The need for a new medical model: a challenge for biomedicine." *Science 196,* 4286, 129–36; and Moira Stewart and Judith Belle Brown (1995) *Patient Centered Medicine: Transforming the Clinical Method.* London: SAGE Publications.

of several major influences that include: the patient's general *health condition* and *will to improve* it, which is particularly observable when it is absent, and depends heavily on the human spirit within; a *place* prepared for care, where responsibilities for other living concerns are reduced to allow the body's natural healing powers to proceed optimally; *nursing care* management of natural bodily processes and prescribed treatments; *medical care* quality, a factor for which the facility and the health system were designed and continually work to improve the collection of attitudes and relationships of *people close to and important* to the patient, often referred to as a support system; and finally, an *uncontrollable power* that is beyond all of us put together. No human being or team of them is ever in control of outcomes. We can influence them for better or worse, but the outcome always remains beyond our actual control. Spiritual caregivers work at providing an interpersonal context that emphasizes that element of healing.

During most of the 1970s my father coped quite functionally with his late-life-onset diabetes and his atherosclerosis and coronary heart failure, keeping its observable manifestations mostly hidden from me and my two older sisters. Our mother had died at 54, 17 years earlier. On his 71st birthday Dad suffered a heart attack while fishing with me on Lake Superior. A three-week rehab stint at a small northern Wisconsin hospital shielded his gradual deterioration until his declining urine output precipitated his transfer 60 miles to a larger city hospital in northern Minnesota. There it became quickly clear to a consulting nephrologist that it wasn't his kidneys that were the problem. His heart was not able to sustain his organ functioning enough for him to continue living. He was at his end.

The cardiologist there asked my sisters and me if he could insert a new device called a Swan Ganz catheter into his heart. He said it would help staff monitor his heart output and evaluate the effect of my dad's medications. I asked him if it would help my dad. "No," he said. I was grateful for his honesty. We said no to its use. There was clearly no more medical influence for Dad. He died there two days later. Nobody on this planet could stop it.

The inherently uncontrollable nature of hospitalization outcomes causes virtually anybody immersed in healthcare culture to experience in some measure an underlying impression of heightened human vulnerability. For patients it begins at admission or a bit before, when a sense of alarm affects the soul enough to motivate the drive to a facility or the phone call for help. That subtle or vivid patient sensation of vulnerability ebbs and flows with every doctor visit, every new prescription, every ruminative moment, every new treatment and every different evaluation of what is already being tried. Hospitals teem with that edge of intermittent hope intertwining with scientific information. Patients feel it far more boldly than experienced clinicians and staff members. But it affects all people involved, some severely, as compassion fatigue, burnout, and repeated trauma exposure statistics show (e.g. Mathieu 2007).

What both patients and staff members do with this pervasive underlying vulnerability can be seen, in human terms, as their unique individual spiritualties. The highly practical concept of spirituality used in this book is *all that people have learned to do, believe, ponder, and practice in order to cope with and enjoy what human beings cannot control*.[3] Essentially one's unique spirituality is what he or she does with her vulnerability in facing the uncontrollable reality that makes up human living.[4] It is the essence of what Atul Gawande has described so richly as "being mortal" (Gawande 2014). It stands at the core of healing.

I learned about this practical understanding of spirituality by working for a decade in a treatment program for addicts that was based solidly on working with the Twelve Steps of Alcoholics Anonymous (AA), not merely learning about them. It became clear to patients who seriously

---

3   The author's definition of spirituality emerged largely from his experience of addressing addicts midway through treatment in "Step Two and Three" groups regarding what they find to rely on for sobriety after acknowledging from their core that they cannot manage their addiction by themselves ("Step One").

4   Even the etymology of the word "control" implies its limitations. The word emerged from the act of stopping the normal rolling movement of something (Latin *contra* meaning "against," with *rotulus*, "a small wheel"). It implies strong but temporary influence without complete command.

engaged with the treatment process that their efforts at staying sober were essential but not sufficient. Nobody could quit drinking for them and they had already learned with years of trying that they couldn't do it by themselves. They began to collaborate with counselors and with one another in ways they never had before. Recovery, the AA word for healing, not only requires spiritual perspectives, it is itself a spiritual process (Kurtz 2010 [1979]).[5] So is dying, and navigating the final path towards it.

In that program I got to see how AA meetings are largely made up of telling and retelling the incredibly open stories of their finding and working with their vulnerability in the face of their own powerlessness over a simple chemical substance as a way to a normal life (Thomsen 1975).[6] One could say that alcoholics who had sought cure for half their lives learned that there is a lifestyle of ongoing healing that one can live without cure. It is rather a way of living with a chronic illness that allows normal experience with a different richness than one could have imagined. It involves as a major component the telling of the key stories of one's struggles, intense regrets, and victories of life.

The sorting out of what can be done to influence a medical outcome from what is beyond us all is eventually a practitioner function in every hospital patient's case. Leaving out of the medical record comments

---

5   In a letter to Bill Wilson responding to his request for help with his intensely frustrating alcoholic debility, Carl Jung suggested that nothing would help him, not even psychoanalysis, except a major spiritual transformation.

6   What set the AA movement apart from others in history and made it so incredibly successful was a radical, extended kind of surrender, the same step all physicians eventually need to take about their patients in general, especially near their time of dying. Nothing effective happens in establishing even a temporary recovery without a radical beginning in authentic and soulful surrender, the first of the well-known, elusive Twelve Steps. After years of blind denial and then more years of earnestly trying to live without alcohol, the original groups almost miraculously found that only their stark admission that alcohol is a greater power than them allowed them to begin a new way of living that didn't include use of it. That new way of living was eventually called recovery, and was characterized by progressive open acknowledgement of shared mutual vulnerability. It allowed victims of alcoholism to stay sober, still only one day at a time. That process stands as a model of living with life's inherent vulnerability that tends to get integrated by hospitalization.

about a patient's established unique individual spirituality neglects some of the most important data in helping that person heal.

There is a long history of the inevitable tension between tangible help and intangible realities, between science-based practice on the one hand and spirituality—along with its far narrower component religion—on the other. That history can be briefly summarized this way.

Spiritual perspectives augment medical and nursing care

Physicians generally know that many if not most of their patients have significant behavioral issues that impede their health, issues that as medical doctors they cannot address effectively. Beleaguered by the demands of administrators, the seemingly useless strictures of funding companies, and the excessive expectations of society, they remain dedicated to their practice. That requires they must leave those complex personal and interpersonal issues to other caregivers. In addition, physicians experience the inadequacy of those other disciplines and systems set up to address the complex and difficult sabotaging issues of a majority of people. Regarding spiritual perspectives, they are mostly confused by religion and quickly abandon it as useful in their work. The one professional chaplain they see for every 90 physicians may not be very competent in understanding and appreciating the culture of medical practice.

Hyper-complex phenomena like human health cannot be understood adequately from one perspective. The word derives from Latin *per* meaning 'through' combined with *specere* meaning 'to look carefully through'. That word developed in order to capture and share the experience of looking at something through something else. We all look at things through our own frameworks of understanding in order to see whatever we see and know whatever we know. Professionals function from very sophisticated perspectives, frames of reference with which to get bits of clarity about what's needed by somebody in obvious pain or in barely observable difficulty. The complex phenomenon of healing requires several of these well-developed perspectives, none of them being in any way perfect.

Let us imagine how the helping disciplines of medicine, nursing, and spiritual leadership all arose and have evolved to their current distinctive practices. Releasing ourselves from the strictures of pages of facts and probable theories, let us back off our characteristic analysis and tune in to our intuition. Where did these professions and their widely differing perspectives on human helping come from? What follows results mostly from imagination and intuition based on a few scientific facts.

They emerged from the same roots—primitives responding to the early emergence of empathy within their evolving minds. Over centuries of trying to help one another with the horrible and unpredictable encroachment of such tragic occurrences as illness, traumatic injuries, foraging failures, birth malformation, enduring disabilities, and death, some patterns of care developed. Vague empathic urges of early human leaders led to all manner of exploration of what could help, from shamanic rituals, utterances and words, rhythms and chants, kind gestures, plants and potions, and whatever else was recollected to have seemed to work from the remembered experience of many generations before.

A highly confusing conglomeration of helping modalities over hundreds of centuries gradually clustered themselves into three that became roughly distinct: 1) direct and immediate assistance with comfort and functions of daily life (nursing); 2) remembering what substances and actions had actually helped bodies heal in the past (medicine); and 3) imploring the overwhelming, mysterious powers beyond the human (religion). For hundreds of millennia they all evolved adjacent to one another, often mixed within the same practitioner, developing in their separate ways, sometimes conflicting and rarely collaborating.

Then Hippocrates and his followers began to pull those disciplines apart in the fourth century BC. They separated clinical practices that relied on direct observation and collecting histories, from those based in belief, ritual, and efforts to influence gods—sharply consolidating the distinction between doctors on the one hand and priests and shamans on the other. With Hippocrates, those two healthcare disciplines, one based in science and the other based in belief, had been separated and their distinctly evolving directions set.

Nursing may have begun first however. We can imagine that it was born in a cave on a day tens of thousands of years ago as one mother felt a twinge of what would eventually be called empathy for a younger mother she saw struggling to care for an infant in very difficult circumstances. She moved to help, initiating what is now the most trusted profession. Ways of helping one another when hurt, sick, or overwhelmed with other natural difficulties evolved informally until Florence Nightingale's insight, writing and organizational gifts brought it to a true profession of its own during and after the Crimean War of the 1850s (Hamilton 2015). (See "Spiritual need and caregiver satisfaction" below.)

After Hippocrates, medicine and religion traveled different paths, as places of care developed from homes and monasteries into hospitals (Slavicek 2012). The two distinct helping methods wrangled considerably as to which way was more "true." Then, during the scientific revolution of the 16th and 17th centuries, the accelerating development of science began to dominate healthcare culture. Pastors and all other religious leaders eventually found very little place for themselves in hospitals. Spiritual perspectives were then left mostly to churches and the very end of life when medicine's role tended to diminish rapidly. Even in the majority of hospitals founded and supported by religious communities, physicians quite completely dominated the culture. The two have remained mostly separated ever since.

Then in the 20th century new modes of caring burst forth that have now begun a gradual *rapprochement* between medicine and spiritual care. In the evolutionary development of addiction treatment, hospice, and palliative care, some clinicians discovered that serious engagement of spiritual perspectives was often essential to real healing processes. It was becoming clear in small circles that at least for some serious conditions, holistic healing could not be practiced well without humanistic consideration of spiritual points of view.

For patients, however, hospitals have always been places where medical practice and spiritual experiences intertwine. Though the organizational structure of healthcare systems is designed to control and cure, people inherently know that in reality all of that eventually fails. The wheels of life roll on. Doctors as the leaders of the treatment processes rub up against their limitations in the stark reality that all patients ultimately get worse and die. Underlying cognizance of that does not wait in patients' minds until they approach death. It plays on patients and their family members all along the way, from eruption of symptoms to admission and waiting for diagnosis until actual death, and for family members for years after that in the profound experience we now call grief.

Researchers continue to confirm the benefits of spiritual care in hospitals, bit by bit and study by study (Flanelly *et al.* 2011; Fitchett and Nolan 2016). But we need to remember that scientific exploration of what works spiritually parallels the perpetual development of medical practice. Further exploration of the results of both medicine and spiritual care in quality research is continuous and, as far as we can see, unending. A few key elements of what was "best practice" in medicine a year ago is now obsolete. Similarly, there is no likelihood that spiritual care research will somehow finally confirm the value of it or define a lasting theory of such care as if it were another invaluable pharmaceutical.

Medicine and spiritual care are parallel perspectives on the healing of people. They both function as partially effective and complementary to one another. Science carries a ring of certainty that belies the fact that medicine remains a human endeavor, always more an art than a science. Like Mulder and Scully in *The X-Files*, or male and female people, science and spirituality augment one another when at their best, never fusing together and neither one being completely effective by itself. Like railroad tracks or human hands, they remain totally distinct from one another, as together they sometimes accomplish great things while never actually joining.

Today, patients' experiences of their clinicians often include impressions of physicians and even busy nurses, in their vague rumblings of ultimate concern, having neither time nor interest. Pastors likewise easily miss the depth of patients' hospitalization experience, possessing neither medical literacy nor interpersonal skills to elicit and hear what transpires inside those troubled souls. Hospice, palliative care, and the clinical ministry movement are making great but still patchy headway in changing that long-standing situation. It is already clear to some that clinical chaplaincy working in those services has a key place in bridging the gap between the views of spirituality and medicine, two endeavors that will likely always remain in creative tension.

A primary feature of clinical chaplaincy has been its dedicated focus on emotion and its primary intervention of persistent conveyed empathy. Since its inception in the 1920s, clinical ministry educators have focused doggedly on helping students to keep at least one eye on what the patient is feeling at any given time, to facilitate further conversation about emotion-ridden disclosures, artfully convey empathy, and continue to follow subsequent emotions, stories, and attitudes that emerge when a person feels deeply understood. As physicians and nurses keep a focus on what a patient says and knows, skilled chaplains rather favor what the patient feels and how that throws light on the essential meanings they place on their current situation. Chaplains elicit patients' inner and often submerged thoughts and attitudes by hearing them talk from their own point of view rather than answering clinicians' questions about what they need to hear.

There was no hospice or palliative care when physicians found cancer in my mother's cervix when she was 52. In the early 1960s, radium implants, barium treatments, and new pain medications like Darvon only dragged her through two years of painful, fruitless treatment. Then I got a call in my junior year of college. My oldest sister ordered me home, even insisting that I take my first plane ride rather than hitchhike the 90 miles for Mom's last days. A priest chaplain was there for several minutes during the final day. I don't think he said anything. Thirty years later I met him at a family funeral and found out why. He had nothing to say. Mom had received the Catholic anointing at home months earlier. The priest chaplain was a kind old man who like many hospital chaplains of that era was unable to relate on a human-to-human level. Without a sacramental role he could only be present. I appreciated his presence and had felt no yearning for him to speak or do anything else. I was glad he was there.

Hospital chaplains and other spiritual caregivers have come a long way since she died in apparent terror, though many are still scurrying to find the competence needed to participate integrally in hospice and palliative care services. The integration of competent spiritual caregivers into healthcare has a long way to go. But it is evolving. Care of the human spirit is still better than it was for Mom. Maybe if she died today someone could have helped her with whatever put that last horrified look on her face.

A brief but pointed perspective on the human spirits of patients, when available in a hospital unit, actually serves as a human basis for other clinicians' work. In some ways it sets the stage for what all other clinicians add to goals of care and treatment regimens. It holds on deftly but stubbornly to the practice of patient-as-person first.

Meeting in the spirituality that is humanism

Healthcare culture at its most basic level functions as beautifully humanistic in the best sense of the word. In their ordinary day-to-day care, members of IDTs come together in a teeming organism of nitty-gritty, here-and-now dedication to humanity. Regardless of any greed, gridlock, and exploitation one finds in various levels of healthcare systems, in the nursing units where direct patient care is taking place, where people are actually caring for people, humanism rules. In emergency care this may be seen most boldly. Staff members temporarily set aside their issues at home and their interpersonal conflicts with one another. They delay the rest they frequently need, shelve their prejudices, and ignore for a time any tightly held life resentments while they engage vigorously in a rare form of decisive, egalitarian care for any human that shows up in medical need. It may be that only policemen and soldiers[7] can rival that vigor of active humanistic bent.

Stories of heroes and heroic events almost invariably appeal to a humanistic core in all of us. We possess an evolving inclination to simply help one another, in spite of the cultural, ethnic, language, and sexual differences, and their related biases, that often cover over our altruistic essence. The impulse to care for fellow humans survives and thrives even amidst the self-absorbed hedonism and egoistic greed that seems to pervade societies for periods of time that seem way too long. Stories of unexpected helping of others arise almost everywhere there is intense human pain and suffering. The 9/11 Twin Tower attacks, hurricane disasters, tsunami calamities, and multi-state electrical grid failures serve as dramatic sources of such stories. Even combat situations sometimes spawn stories of unexpected bursting forth of soldiers' deep reverence for humanity, including that of the enemy.[8] At our core we are all more similar than different.

The medical record offers a major location for physicians, nurses, and spiritual caregivers to meet in the endeavor of humanistic care. Medicine, nursing, social work, and spirituality are all characterized by traditional devotion to humanism, dedication of considerable focused energy towards each individual person and the human community as a whole. All of these disciplines are, at their core, deeply humanistic. That similarity grounds the potential for collaboration, which upon reflection can play out effectively in the hospital medical record.

Institutional spiritual care, or pastoral care as it is still sometimes known, also carries a strong humanistic character that is generally more obvious and earthy than the words and deeds of leaders of organized religion. The formative chaplain education of certified chaplains has

---

7   Including all military personnel to the extent that they are exposed to combat or near combat experience.
8   A few memorable movies that carry this theme include *The Enemy Below* (1957) and *Warhorse* (2011).

long emphasized a humanistic perspective. Clinical pastoral education (CPE),[9] which spawned the clinical ministry movement (see Hall 1992; Hemenway 1996; King 2007) beginning in the 1920s, flourishes largely through groups focusing on verbatim reports of individual patient care conversations, centering carefully on what any given patient needs rather than what is either "right" or superior theologically. CPE and certified professional chaplaincy continue to provide and teach spiritual care practices with a major humanistic emphasis.

Formative education is only now, in its evolutionary development, beginning to foster substantive and useful spiritual care charting. Only a few CPE programs beckon budding spiritual caregivers into the wisdom of stating in writing spiritual needs in common terms that everyone can not only understand but see and hear in present human interactions. Attention to what pastoral care students write in the medical record has only recently begun preparing them to meet their medical and nursing colleagues in representing patients' spiritual and personal issues they discover in their conversations with them. That budding practice is beginning to fill a hole in medical recordkeeping. As Atul Gawande (2014, p.151) has written, "Our most cruel failure in how we treat the sick…is the failure to recognize that they have priorities beyond merely being safe and living longer; that the chance to shape one's story is essential to sustaining meaning in life."

Spiritual caregivers who want to better integrate themselves into the humanistic and pragmatic hospital culture can benefit highly from learning to focus on the *human spirit* of patients and families at least as much as they think in terms of theological concepts like the Holy Spirit, salvation, and forces of the universe. Helpful as some of these concepts may be in some circles, they generally fall flat on the ears and eyes of IDT members. Contenting ourselves with language about God and church while ignoring the human spirit only isolates us from the medical culture in which we are working.

Use of the term *human spirit* not only serves effectively for staff communication, but it accurately describes people's challenges and

---

9   See the Association for Clinical Pastoral Education website www.ACPE.edu

dilemmas. After all, it is the human spirit that brings a patient to healthcare facilities in the first place, as it becomes unsettled enough from a worsening medical issue to motivate the seeking of help. It is the human spirit that becomes "pressed down" in what is commonly called depression. It is the human spirit that becomes riled against the limitations of life that we will never understand in the emotional phenomenon we call grief from searing, unstoppable losses. It is the human spirit that is wounded forever in childhood abuse by one of the parental authorities we painfully and persistently yearned to have on our side as children and seriously troubled adults.

As a result of their history, nursing, medicine, and clinical chaplaincy take very different and complementary approaches to meeting the human spirit of patients. Their listening is so distinct from one another that we actually need three different words for those types of listening.[10] Physicians need specific information to diagnose and treat so they focus listening on what they need to know in *diagnostic* listening. Nurses listen for patients' concrete needs for comfort and their attitudes about self-care, compliance with treatment regimens, and overall health in *immediate concrete* listening. Chaplains and spiritually interested clinicians seek to create a context in which patients can talk freely from their own point of view about whatever is affecting their spirit on the deepest levels, in *personal* listening. Different as they are from one another, they form a necessary triumvirate of holistic care, and all of these caregivers occasionally enter significantly into one another's primary listening styles. Optimally, the combined relevant results can form a human picture of each patient in the medical record.[11]

Spiritual care chart entries that contain brief stories or descriptions of the complex and difficult human situations in which patients find themselves are still often seen as counter-cultural in healthcare settings.

---

10   The listening we do at home with lovers and spouses and in the workplace with colleagues are also distinct.

11   All three make assessments as part of their role so to some degree they all listen diagnostically. All are human beings so they all have their moments of personal listening. And in crisis times all may be pulled into the immediate need for concrete listening that doesn't miss the emergency.

Exception-based charting,[12] electronic medical records, evidence-based practices, and the current trend towards gathering research data seem to have further reduced the perceived relevance of such notes. But chart entries that honor and convey the deep humanity and uniqueness of every individual also support those caregivers who insist on honoring the humanness of patients, a perspective that can easily slip from view in some IDT members' fierce dedication and hurried decisiveness.

Shared patient narratives keep teams human

Hearing stories that convey a patient's humanness, even second hand, in the medical record tends to keep some warmth in clinicians' impressions of their patients (Gottshall 2013). It has been shown that our first impressions of people focus on how we see two aspects of a person who is new to us: competence and warmth (Cuddy 2015). Both are essential to developing rapport between people. We instinctively wonder, "Can I trust that this stranger is competent in what she is purporting to do?" and, "Does she convey at least a hint of genuine warmth?" indicating that she really sees me as a person. Human narratives promote a truly human impression, contributing to an overall promotion of care throughout an entire hospital unit culture.

The process of becoming a clinician necessarily makes emotions secondary to thinking, judgement, memory, and decisive agency. The term "clinician" itself is derived from the Greek *klinikos*, literally meaning "from the bed." That etymology suggests that somebody noticed over the centuries that when something tragic happens, high emotion is not what is called for. The sick or injured one needs a bed at those times because she is at least unsteady on her feet. It is no time for hysteria in bystanders, not even for inquiry about one's current feeling life. What is needed is somebody who is knowledgeable, skilled, and can remain objective enough to make useful decisions. The common use of the term "clinical" as implying "coldly dispassionate" emerged from overextension of that earlier use.

---

12   A style of medical record-keeping that only allows entering what is different from the established protocol about this patient.

Still, humor, irreverence, wit, and either raucous or stifled laughter have long been staples of the coping skills of healthcare professionals. Human stories bring people together, mostly unconsciously. Warmth in stories about a patient's appearance, mannerisms, lifestyle, or unique communication patterns brings most people involved into a common arena of human foibles and shared imperfections. Austere analysis and strident cogitation can only last for so long before the need for emotional connection rises involuntarily. Colorful patient stories, from them or about them, add to that common, humanistic staff spirituality.

The rapid rise of palliative care programs has boldly illustrated the need for practitioners to tune in to what is happening in patients' *souls*, that largely mysterious energizing core of any person. Patients' own stories of their health experience—impressions of the varied staff caring for them; their developing attitudes about their current condition and prognosis; their feelings of trepidation and spindly hope; concerns about payment, pets, and employment; worries about temporary or even permanent disability; and repetitive thoughts about whatever soulful concerns they're leaving at home—actually help shape the remainder of their lives. And as the hospice movement has shown, there is an additional value of this verbal processing for patients whose medical condition is deteriorating, to disclose and converse about the deeper end-of-life issues that eventually descend upon us all.

Serious healthcare concerns affect our core. Facing them shapes our lives and teaches us about ourselves (Frank 2013 [1995]). Physical healthcare events will likely always remain times of gaining perspective on the unavoidable limitations of human resilience. They are times of realization, making real the helplessness we constantly live with and that we ordinarily keep ourselves from feeling as we strive to maintain a measure of comfort in ordinary, everyday living. They are times of facing the inevitable while holding on to what is left of us, enhancing that remaining spark of liveliness to the greatest extent possible, living as well as we can, and eventually dying as beautifully as possible. Sharing patient stories enhances that entire process, for both patients and staff members.

Spiritual need and caregiver satisfaction

The experience called the "helper's high," recognized by caregivers for hundreds of years, has been shown to improve job and life satisfaction in many cases (Luks 2001).[13] Despite long-standing efforts to make human responses secondary in clinicians' formative education in order to enhance objectivity, virtually all practitioners are affected emotionally by some of their patients' conditions and unique predicaments. They are compelled to respond warmly and more kindly to some particular people than to others, as unpredictably as falling in love. But it naturally feels good to help people in need and it unsettles us to fail at that effort. It enhances practitioners' work and career satisfaction to respond to the identified needs of patients.[14] Some of those needs can be seen as spiritual.

The often vague awareness of a lack of something for which one yearns, consciously or unconsciously, can be called spiritual need. Sometimes the human spirit just aches, for reasons that are cumulative and only vaguely understood. Humans naturally seek peace, serenity, and enthusiasm for satisfactory living. When that tranquility seems elusive or unattainable, we feel a need for something that will bring it back. We may not even know what that remedy may be. For purposes of addressing the inner struggles that accompany healthcare challenges, we can define spiritual needs broadly as *unpleasant or painful experiences of having difficulty finding meaning and purpose relative to what we cannot control.*

---

13   The "helper's high" was first described by Allan Luks, who surveyed thousands of volunteers across the United States and found that people who reached out to other people consistently stated that their health improved when they started to volunteer. About half reported experiencing a "high" feeling; 43 percent felt stronger and more energetic; 28 percent experienced a sensation of inner warmth; 22 percent felt calmer and less depressed; 21 percent experienced greater feelings of self-worth, and 13 percent experienced fewer aches and pains.

14   It is questionable, however, whether clinicians who merely "have a job" or a healthcare role, or those who over-focus on remuneration and financial perks actually benefit spiritually as much from their helping as those whose practice is more authentically altruistic.

That definition is intentionally expansive, inclusive of needs of varying intensity on a scale from vague yearnings to tortuous life binds. Spiritual needs go unmet most of the time, physically parallel to natural bodily aches and pains in aging or wishes and daydreams in childhood. A simple example is the need to verbally share what is deeply affecting us—with someone.

Empathy almost defines the story of Florence Nightingale's contribution to nursing, and it was spiritual need that precipitated her passion for helping. Feisty, outspoken, and uncommonly assertive for her historical period, she was nonetheless motivated by human compassion for untreated and neglected soldiers during a stint near combat lines of the Crimean War. Nursing practice had existed informally since humanity lived in caves, but took a quantum leap ahead with her empathic realization of the prolonged suffering alone of wounded young men.

Historically there had always been compassionate women and a few men assisting people with the immediate physical needs and human spirit challenges that accompanied physical trauma. But there on a single occasion, when Nightingale ambled through a large military infirmary, the filthy conditions of overcrowding and intense needs for the fundamentals of life—clean water, fresh air, healthful food and basic sanitation—a moment of realization inspired her dedication to improving those conditions as they spurred her into a passionate mission lasting for the rest of her life. Those young men's physical needs were being exacerbated by inner suffering that sliced through her composure, found her heart and moved her soul. She saw them silently crying out for a caring presence and a bit of physical comfort as much as for medical help (Hamilton 2015). She was responding to their spiritual needs, as that moment grew into what is now the world's most trusted profession. Recognized spiritual need has always been at the heart of nursing.

Nurse practitioner Anne Butler[15] tells a simple story that illustrates how easily even intense spiritual needs can remain submerged. She believes the story is repeated, albeit in less dramatic terms, hundreds of times a day in hospice and intensive care situations.

A man on her palliative care practice was obviously in his last hours. She entered his room minutes after a chaplain had left him. The chaplain had written in the chart, "Patient appears quite disturbed and declining my invitation to offer a prayer. No need for further visit at this time."

Having been treating the man for his pain, Anne read the note and approached the patient with an intuitive probing observation. Noting his facial expression as intent and anxious, she easily guessed that an element of his anxiety was either interpersonally or personally spiritual[16] rather than medical. "I sense that you have something to tell me," she said. Nodding vigorously he struggled to say, "I want to tell you what I have loved and what I will miss before I let go." She then proceeded to elicit from him his tearful sharing about three treasured cows he had raised from birth and nurtured for years on his farm, including his vivid expression of his soulful affection for them. Who would care for them now? How could he abandon them? When she astutely asked, "Did you name them?" he broke into tears. "Lazy Daisy, Buttercup and Lollipop," he said.

Can there be any doubt that in telling that story, which had been lying just below the surface of his awareness, he had made use of her help to consolidate a bit of healing that helped him die more peacefully? The chaplain had missed the story that was bursting to be told. It was the palliative care medical person who listened personally. Clearly, from a humanist point of view, the man's need for "telling" can be seen as a spiritual one. His human spirit was crying out to share it. Anne's heart was lifted a bit forever by eliciting that story's telling, hearing it, and retelling it many times.

---

15   Once a palliative care practitioner at George Washington University Hospital and then practicing in Greenville, SC.

16   See Chapter 2.

Among the reasons to focus care on spiritual needs and record them is simply that IDT members feel better when they recognize spiritual needs or hear about how they have been at least addressed by someone, as a part of a person's hospitalization. Over the length of a career, meeting spiritual needs increases a practitioner's life satisfaction. Describing a patient in her unique personhood in the medical record helps bring a human-to-human tone to all the caring interactions of the staff. Identifying *specific* spiritual needs, however, in brief but concrete detail, calls out a bit more focused empathy from anyone reading that description. A chart note comment, for example, stating that a chaplain listened to a patient and supported him, will likely be passed over easily as generalized and redundantly patterned. A more concrete one, artfully disclosing within the limits of confidentiality, that the patient vented significant resentments and regrets, will more likely strike home to the reader. A further, even more explicit comment, that he shared a painful yearning for personal contact with an estranged relative, will be more likely felt by IDT members, with a bit of satisfaction that a personal or interpersonal need is being addressed.

In this broad and pragmatic sense of spiritual need, hospitals are filled with them. When the top leadership of hospitals like Massachusetts General begin their mission statement, "Guided by the needs of our patients..." it is likely they do not realize very clearly the spiritual needs, the inner turmoil, that physical needs create. But very often those needs are disturbing somewhere on a range from merely disquieting annoyances or mild apprehensions to uniquely excruciating twists of life.

Sorting religion's sustaining power from its destructive peril

It has long been known in common culture that only a small fraction of what is spiritual is to be found in churches and religious practice. Yet real religion remains strong in a majority of the world's people and religious needs often lie dormant in patients until probed. It is in difficult times such as hospitalization that what one has partially learned from religious lore is reflexively sought in efforts to bolster the human spirit. Anyone hoping to act sensitively to religious needs will be wise to appreciate both the value and the peril of religion in the lives of hospitalized people.

Wally Peterson was a Lutheran clinical pastoral educator who developed coronary heart failure in his 30s. Long before his death at 43, he was once hospitalized in intensive care for several weeks. Afterwards he was recounting his experience there as a member of a colleague panel assembled to share similar stories of personal trials. A few of his words have stayed with me in the decades since:

> In those weeks when I didn't know if I would live or die that day, I was not sustained much by my family who did come to see me, nor by my colleagues who were steeped in caregiving skills. In those days what held me together was, "Now I lay me down to sleep; I pray the Lord my soul to keep. If I should die before I wake, I pray the Lord my soul to take," and "Jesus loves me this I know, 'cuz the Bible tells me so."

This academically educated and thoroughly trained professional found that childhood religious sentiment returned when he needed memories of it most.

Some spiritual needs are religious. That simply means that some efforts to meet uncontrollable life are related to the established traditions of the world's great faith groups. Besides such common human spiritual needs as guilt, dying, and discouragement, other complex and intense needs are directly related to religious belief and practice. It is the collected body of formational and inspirational stories that feeds people most and motivates them to practices and beliefs that enrich their lives. The power of those stories is largely lost in the transformations that occur in the religious teachings that follow after the founders' deaths. Those fundamental changes result from the human tendency to over-focus on control, reducing reverence for transcendence and creating a factual literalism that has repeatedly split and splintered the world's great religions and created aspects of them that can become highly destructive to the human spirit.

Where did religion come from? From a humanist point of view, in the evolution of helping, a few great spiritual innovators emerged. They were men and women who became leaders because they possessed uncommon abilities to incorporate stories, conceptualize beliefs, create practices, and establish rituals that were successful in helping people retain resilience and a bit of calm in facing transcendence, that awe experience of being jolted by sensing something that is obviously incomprehensible. They were fine humanists who cared about people deeply and worked, thought, taught, and lived to improve people's experience of the uncontrollable world. They were a small class of individuals that includes some whose names we all recognize—Moses, Muhammad, Jesus, Gautama Buddha—and a few others with whom we may not be familiar, whose influence has lived for centuries. Most of the eight billion people on this planet still revere at least one of them and have benefited by that leader's life and what he or she left behind.

Today people variously turn to spiritual beliefs and traditional religious practices during healthcare challenges. For some the anxiety of hospitalization intensifies their religious convictions and sometimes the rigidity and relative contextual incognizance that can accompany them. For others, critical thinking and negative experiences of religion had already prompted exclusion of religious or even spiritual beliefs from consideration when making their healthcare decisions. Still others, like Wally Peterson, resurrect concepts and beliefs that they had partially incorporated during their childhood development, seeking for any effective meaning that might sustain them in this life–death challenge.

For the purpose of practical patient care, religion here means *a body of thinking, practice, and teaching organized by people to assist the human spirit in ways related to the established traditions of the world's great religions.* As we have said, an individual's spirituality is the unique array of ways that a person deals with the uncontrollable. Religion on the other hand, refers to organized individual or communal activity intended to enhance one's human spirit. For practical purposes, one could say that as school is to an education, religion is to spirituality. The difficulty is that religion has clearly not always been beneficial to either the human spirit or to the human community.[17]

Seen from the pragmatic and humanistic perspective of clinical practice, the massive phenomenon of religion has two faces: solid supportive grounding for resilience in hard times on the one hand, and truncating rigidity with a tendency towards abusive exploitation on the other. Religious convictions held rigidly lose their humanitarian roots. Failures of religion are everywhere. That is the way of evolution— innumerable failures, new strains, dead ends, breakthrough mutations, and the halting, tortuous spread of "the new" across the planet. In that process, religion's negative strains—exploitation, domination, oppression, coercion, and even wars based on beliefs held far too certainly—make the inherent human vulnerability from an uncontrollable world worse. Indeed there seems to be a phenomenon called religious addiction characterized by such excessive devotion to one religious ideology that such a zealot has difficulty appreciating the human condition and what is best for a person overall. It is especially destructive when the religious addict becomes a leader, and when an entire sect systemically supports destructive religion. Seen from a humanist point of view, religiosity is not always benign.

What is seen now in the clinical setting is a complex conglomeration of the latest evolutionary phase of religious development mixed with residual damage from religious failure. Anyone caring for the human spirit there will often be compelled to distinguish between the best and worst of religion. The best sustains, inspires, and guides. The worst—scary complexity of religious belief and practice, along with its confusion, half-learned principles, failed observances, backsliding regrets, alarming after-life fears, and vague yearnings for a clear conscience—poses a formidable task for spiritual care.

---

17   Neither is a person's spirituality. That phenomenon will be taken up in Chapter 3.

That is why the religious area of spirituality will, for the foreseeable future, need well prepared religious leaders to hear the unique spiritual struggles and binds of even minimally religious patients, understand critically, and respond as effectively as possible. The history of thinking and terminology of religion remains esoteric and even senseless to most clinicians. In vital situations they sometimes find that religious beliefs, values, and practices can loom strong in deciding about optimum medical care. But wisely, they mostly decline to engage that aspect of human culture due to the complexity of its issues and the power of its persuasion over many individuals. Indeed, anyone who dares to chart spiritual care ought to possess some measure of confidence and competence wading around in the hyper-complexity that is today's mixture of religious teaching and myriad spiritual perspectives, both traditional and contemporary. Clinicians and other IDT members sometimes need wisdom from a caregiver who understands specific aspects of religious practice of various kinds, and is able to sort the wheat from the chaff of any given patient. Chapter 4 of this book deals directly with religious issues common to hospital patients.

A humanist caregiver approach, although possibly non-religious philosophically, does not ignore religion. Some religious needs are deeply spiritual and highly relevant to patient care. For example, Catholic, Muslim, Native American, Hindu, and Buddhist rituals for numerous reasons can generate fierce patient and family insistence on those needs being met. Quiet resentments, vocal complaints, or acting-out conflict result if no attempt is made to at least address them. Much of the world's theology was fashioned around the reality that we all die and nobody really knows what happens next. Concern about "eternal salvation" can quickly emerge among family members as being at stake for a patient, even when that patient has ignored religious practices for decades. On the other hand, a spiritual caregiver who contents himself with making religious remarks and rituals, ignoring the broader aspect of spirituality, generally becomes irrelevant to IDT staff and most patients. When a given religious affiliation is recorded, the level of importance the person places on that religion is best explored and recorded as well (Puchalski and Romer 2000).[18]

Writing concisely about a patient's religious history, beliefs and practice in the medical record can, on important occasions, help those caregivers who read it to better understand that patient in her values, attitudes, assumptions, convictions, practices, and other personality aspects that shape her ethical and other treatment decisions. Mere reference to a patient's religious affiliation, however, offers little insight into that person's unique human spirit and current spirit needs. To write that the person is an affiliated Methodist, an American Buddhist, or a lapsed Catholic means little without reference or story that indicates what that means now to this particular individual.

The spiritual content of a patient conversation includes anything that impinges substantively on the human spirit of that person, and especially what relates to the reason for hospitalization. A broad framework of understanding spirituality that guides listening far beyond religious practice, heritage, and current beliefs, is necessary to make observations and comments about the current state of patients' human spirits. Chapter 2 lays out one such humanist framework that serves as an example of a theory of spirituality that honors the depth and breadth of all that either buoys or sinks the human spirit of hospitalized people.

---

18 In the FICA tool designed at George Washington University the "I" stands for the "importance" religion holds for a given person. ("F" is "faith," "C" is "community" relationships supporting or hindering the patient's life, and "A" is how the patient wants staff to "address" the spiritual aspect of care.)

2

Theory

A Humanist View of Spirituality:
Universal Sources of Patient Stories

Our very selves are perpetually recreated in stories. Stories do not simply describe the self; they are the self's medium of being.

ARTHUR W. FRANK (1995, P.53)

Human stories of personal significance emerge from sources that are common to us all, despite the enormous differences among us. Some aspects of life are experienced by all people everywhere—eating, friendship, sexuality, sickness, and emotionality to name a few. That makes those fundamental themes points of connection between patients and caregivers no matter how diverse their ethnic cultures may be. If the language barrier can be breached, then staff members can connect with almost any patient and family member by eliciting and hearing unstructured stories from what we can call the *primary arenas of the human spirit.*

The enormous scope of spirituality as "all that people have learned to do, believe, ponder, and practice in order to cope with and enjoy what human beings cannot control," is unmanageable without some structure for a spiritual caregiver's listening. Such an organizing framework that can make a patient's spirituality more practicable to communicate about can be made up of phenomenological impressions of what seems to affect the human spirit most on a given day, and during crisis times.

A brief look at one's own typical day offers hints at the aspects of life that tend to touch or disturb the human spirit deeply and often. As you are driving home from work, for example, what are the themes that tend to capture your attention and prod your reflections? Children, if you have them, a current lover, a worrisome bill, a co-worker's rant, a tough case at work, a sick uncle, or a weekend plan, all quietly vie for either brooding attention or action planning. A half dozen of these arenas move in and out of your mind, partially responding to your intentional direction and partly with a life of their own. Some more pervasive issues like seeking a new house or career lie mostly dormant beneath, occasionally bursting into consciousness as well. Why those particular themes? They compel us because they are universal among humanity and they constitute our human spirit lives.

For many years I have asked groups of people one question and spent an hour or so recording their answers on a chalk board. The question is always something like: "What are the aspects of life that feed you the most, the parts that offer fulfilling and lasting satisfaction, and enjoyment of a single day?" When the participants look at the final framework they have created on the board, it is convincing that the same life areas in which we find delight, inspiration and satisfaction are the ones in which we meet our most painful events. Groups to whom I have asked this question have been addicts in treatment, chaplain students, clergy, mental health patients, and mixed gender groups interested in broadly conceived spirituality. The spiritual arenas below have been distilled from those communal conversations.

Rather than our typical assumptions that we are in charge of our own living, we can just as accurately think of ourselves as actually living in a sea of mysteries, phenomena that are never completely comprehended, that we cannot control. We can influence these primary arenas of life but—like our breathing, our affections, and our bodily vigor—we never actually control them. These are not some ethereal fantasies but clusters of real life experience. From outside them we only touch their depth, as in our love lives and our parenting, knowing little about them until we seriously engage in them with lovers and children. Then they continue to unfold endlessly. The words "mystery" and "mist" derive from similar Latin words, both referring to phenomena that are perpetually only known partially. Like objects in a cloud, concerns in these arenas get clearer at times but never become consistently distinct. And it is in the context of each one of these arenas that we find both the most awe-filled beauty and the most jolting tragedies. We can use a framework of these arenas, roughly three dozen of them, as a humanistic listening map for patient stories.

Virtually all human experience contains a spiritual perspective. Upon reflection we easily know that everywhere we look we touch what cannot be controlled but can either delight or sadden us or even drown us in disaster. Spirituality is essentially a constant flow of decisions we cannot escape, about what we can do about our primary concerns and what lies outside our influence. This chapter outlines the primary arenas in which those decisions, many of them reflexive and barely conscious, present themselves to us. Spiritual arenas are broad aspects of life that abide no easy success, no reduction to black and white, and very few simple answers. They plunge us into the most difficult and painful situations we ever encounter. And they can at times rapidly bestow on us joy and unexpected shining success. These arenas are the most common sources of patient stories that emanate from the human core.

Spiritual maturity could be defined as habitually living with generalized acceptance and frequent joyfulness on the edge between the strictures of over-simplifying excessive certainty on the one hand and the overwhelming alarm and anxiety of tragedy on the other, in daily facing an uncontrollable world. The person with a level of spiritual maturity has learned to live in the ambiguity of constant surroundings that she cannot control, having overcome the natural human penchant for doggedly seeking certainty and mastery. Religious dogma, the soulless lawyer, the emotionally clueless physician, and the polarized politician all exemplify the current evolutionary need for more spiritual maturity in many of our societies. Close examination of any of these stuck life deserts would likely show a shallowness in success regarding many of the spiritual arenas described below. A degree of spiritual maturity is required for anyone purporting to care extensively for the spiritual issues and binds of another person.

For purposes of organizational clarity we divide these story themes into clusters taken from four classical divisions of spiritual experience—relationships with oneself, other people, communities, and transcendence. Dividing them this way makes them look deceptively neat and clearly distinct from one another. Actually they intertwine, reinforce, and conflict with one another in complex ways that gratefully do not need to be clarified in order to share current content of them for the benefit of both chart note writer and reader. Some of them, such as major losses and emotional self-care, can actually involve all of the other arenas.

This intersecting and transecting of patients' spiritual arenas is exacerbated by the listener's own stories. A great deal of the clinical educational model used in formative preparation for professional chaplains is aimed at gaining as thorough an understanding of oneself as possible so as to minimize contamination of the patient's stories by unconscious evoking of similar charged stories of the caregiver's own personal history. Improving awareness of this annoying distortion, first called transference/countertransference and projection by Freud, remains a key aspect of becoming and remaining a spiritual clinician, as will be seen in the Epilogue.

When a caregiver with the time and the interest hears a patient mention any of these aspects of life, as named in Table 2.1, it may be time to facilitate further disclosure, stay mostly quiet, listen creatively, authentically care human to human, and decide whether or not there is anything relevant in the conversation to record in the medical record.

Table 2.1 Axis map of primary spiritual arenas
(sources of patient narratives)

Personal spirituality	Interpersonal spirituality	Transcendent spirituality	Communal spirituality
Self-regard	Romantic love	Nature	Family of origin
Physical self-care	Parenting	Losses	Ethnic heritage
Emotional self-care	"Childing"	Mortality	Neighborhood
Work	Friendship	Personal deity	Gender community
Sexuality	Learning	Religion	Peer communities
Development/ aging	Elders	Creativity/arts	Faith community
Materiality	Siblings	Cosmic harmony	Nation
Nesting	Grandparenting		Human community
Athletics/dance	Help giving		
Hobbies	Help getting		

Interpersonal spirituality: Who I love and who loves me

The first cluster of arenas is made up of ten rich yet tragic relationships with other people. It is safe to say that the human spirit is affected on a daily basis by interpersonal relationships at least as much as by anything else. To a great degree evolution has arranged us that way. The processes of reproduction and development compel us into crucial two-person relationships. We all have, or at least had, a mother and a father, relationships that we augment by liaisons with other older men and women. We naturally seek friends and lovers, and we may be treated to and challenged by siblings and our own children. We naturally talk about these relationships that affect our human spirits so profoundly, unless events of our past inhibit that natural sharing. We tend to turn our relational life, the delight and the pain, into stories.

The etymology of the word re-late (Latin *re* meaning "back or again," and *latus* meaning "side") suggests it originally referred to how we humans go back to being beside another person over and over. Experience suggests that we do that because of an affinity that continues to draw us together repeatedly in a unique configuration of seeking consistency in the exchange of comfort, support, and pleasure that we need, despite difficulties and failures that arise between us and that other person.

Our relationships with other people boost and challenge our human spirits many times a day and they do so in profound ways. Dramatic events like hospitalization almost invariably bring a few of those relationships to the fore. The people we hope will pay attention to us when we need medical care become subjects of stories told from our hospital beds. When a patient mentions any of these ten relationships described below, in either positive or negative terms, there is an invitation and at least a minor need for somebody to show interest, to linger, and to hear.

ROMANTIC LOVE STORIES

I remember the seventh-grade (age 12–13 years) moment in which I first noticed the compelling curve of a girl's ankle as I was returning to my seat from sharpening a pencil. Naïve, a bit confused and newly exhilarated, I'd entered the spiritual arena of intimate loving, that brand new chasm of astonishing joy and vexing confusion into which adolescence flings us all. Falling in love and slogging through the changes life brings to both partners in attempting a long-term relationship are highly spiritual, bringing some of the most lofty highs and dismal lows to the human spirit.

The intimate loving arena is one of the most universal and intense. In its typical unforgettable temporary run, the falling in love phase knows the gamut from life-changing ecstasy to the soul-searing pain of jolting loss. Romance inspires and devastates most all humans everywhere. Almost always playing somewhere on everyone's mind, that inscrutable arena is either yearning for, pulled into, or warmed by at least one rich memory of life's greatest joy—being loved sumptuously, emotionally, and carnally in an unexplainable partnership of two treasuring one another. When a patient talks about a romantic partner, the relationship itself, or a divorce, spiritual experience of soul depth lies just below the surface, regardless of how ordinary that conversation may seem.

Love stories persist as compelling tearjerkers and riotous comedies, generation after generation, now embellished by splendid visual media. Romance remains a source of fascinating personal stories for everyone, many of those tales never having been told. Our own most passionate or emotionally romantic ones insert themselves quietly into our memories forever, until an apparently caring face asks something like, "How did you two meet anyway?" or "What went wrong between you two?" Romance fills our human spirit, pushing aside everything else and inspires the creation of most songs that live awhile in popularity. While patients' love stories, past or recent, may not always fit the criteria for inclusion in a chart note, sometimes they do. And noting the interaction between visiting spouses and lovers can bring clues as to how to address some spiritual needs.

Professional chaplains report that care they provide directly to individual interdisciplinary team (IDT) members is largely about their love lives. Some of it is celebrating, most of it is painful. The engagement ring and story enliven any work group for a time. And stark comments like, "What am I gonna do about my husband?" or "You aren't gonna believe what she did/said last night?" invite stories about what isn't flourishing about the love life. Both kinds of stories need to be heard.

During a crisis, one person most of us want present with us and yearn for if they're not is either our committed lover or our truest friend. Sometimes the same person is both.

"CHILDING": STORIES ABOUT ONE'S PARENTS, AT ANY AGE

Barry Manilow's recording of lilting song "Ships" (Arista 1979) paints a sadly realistic picture of a father and son walking on a beach together bearing the discomfort of distance that has always characterized their relationship. The metaphor of ships passing in the night[1] conveys the situation of occasionally being geographically close but souls remaining barely able to connect with the intricacies of one another's direction, richness, and emotionally charged concerns. How we interact with our parents varies considerably among us, but our relationships with them are always fairly charged with warmth and appreciation along with disappointment and frustration. Nowhere do the inabilities to say enough in love and the shades of deepest gratefulness linger together more closely and persistently with frustration and regret than in conversations with our parents at any age.

Walking my dog one night and noticing cracks in a sidewalk, I suddenly realized that I had been moving towards abandoning the Catholic priesthood for over three years. I was unbelievably shocked to realize at that moment that I was actually leaving it. Only moments later I knew I would have to soon tell my dad. He was so proud of me in that role, being a German Catholic all his life, an exceptionally kind and loyal parent, and never having finished 11th grade (age 16–17 years) himself.

It was after dinner at his little widower house. Mom had died 16 years earlier, and I surmise she would have been devastated by my decision. He was doing the dishes at the sink, as I cleared the table. "What would you think if I wouldn't be a priest anymore?" I tendered. He didn't turn around and face me. After a pause he said, "Well, if you think I would love you any less, you're wrong." A father's blessing for our lives will always stand as pivotal.

There are at least dozens of memorable stories about our fathers that when told communally bring laughter, tears, admiration, and also incredible sadness. Our fathers inspire, prod, delight, disappoint, wound, and mold us. They mystify us as we go through life feeling indeed like two ships passing in the night, close but so, so far away.

---

[1]   The phrase "ships that pass in the night" is from Longfellow's poem, "Elizabeth" published in 1883 in *The Courtship of Miles Standish: Elizabeth*, New York: Houghton, Mifflin and Company, p.86.

Mothers are the first "higher powers" we meet. We must contend with them and their limitations from their breast and cuddle to their nursing home and casket. Any story about mom is open to significant depth when probed. It has long been recognized that the relationship with one's parents heavily affects the most basic shaping of the childhood human spirit. Parents color our authority relationships all through life. Whenever we tell stories of our parents we find just a bit more perspective on what our parents were like, how they regarded us, how they contributed to our lives and also how they failed us. Telling those stories tends to reshape our idealizing and mitigate our "awful-izing," bringing them both into a warmer, softer, more realistic light.

The images one develops of one's parents in toddlerhood, childhood, and adolescence take on a hue that can differ widely among our siblings and certainly contrast with how those parents see themselves. It is remarkable how differently from one another siblings remember their parents. Those drastically differing memories demonstrate clearly how our own perceptions of our parents become skewed and distorted. Each of us had a unique relationship with the same parents. Some events that involved us but not our siblings were quickly forgotten by them yet became life bending for us. My sisters never knew that our father didn't do military service because one of his legs was shorter than the other. They never hunted with him nor saw him in the crowd at their basketball games. I don't think they ever really wrestled with him. And they weren't there when he had that eventually fatal heart attack on Lake Superior. At the same time, who knows what they treasure that was just between them and Dad, about which I know nothing. We agree on many things about him, yet each of us has a few of our own stories that exclusively included Dad and each of us alone.

Whether patient stories about their parents are unrealistically glowing or shaded in bitterness, they can be some of the most important stories of all to tell.

PARENTING: STORIES ABOUT ONE'S CHILDREN

Following any phone call from one of my adult children there is a glow that persists for hours. I believe that is normal. Even if the conversation was mostly about a problem or a decision with which I can't agree, communication in depth with one's offspring injects a kind of energy in the soul for which there is no perfect word in English. Pride may be the closest, but remains totally inadequate. Most of us who have parented children can talk endlessly about them once we get started. This is one spiritual arena that usually needs little prodding to initiate conversation about, in any venue from an elevator and a grocery line, to a book club, a hospital bed, and a funeral home—unless one of them has become estranged. That most painful of all relational events hurts too much to talk seriously about.

There is no substitute for time spent with your child. Nobody else can invest that. There are convenience and function substitutes, in *au pairs*, coaches, babysitters, day care workers, and the like. But if for no other reason than to avoid regrets in your later years, quiet time focusing on what is happening in the heart and mind of your offspring has no quality equal. "Eye time" dedicated to the "Hey Dad, look at me!" yearning; "do time" in a shared project of making something together; "with time," such as walking together somewhere or quietly watching a silly cartoon; "lap time," and other "cuddle time" that shares the warmth of your bodies; and "yea time" in which a parent energetically expresses the genuine pride of seeing a kid's success. These times are what feeds the soul of a boy or girl and without enough of them there is yearning, stridency to find parenting eyes, ache for approval, and simply deep lack of "standing with" the man or "sweetness with" the woman from whom you first emerged. There are many who never have the chance to parent an offspring of their own, and many who let the thousands of chances pass them by with distractions from this most important role that anyone ever accepts.

Regrets about one's parenting role, about poor decisions, lamented neglect, and missed moments crucial to your child, veil themselves from Christmas letters and party socializing. But they occasionally slip out to an unsuspecting listener—friend, acquaintance, amicable stranger, or caregiving professional— and that listener can then care for that person's human spirit uniquely. Such moments—worries and misgivings about your offspring—when they are disclosed in a hospital, belong in summary form in the medical record in some form because they speak to the current state of that human spirit. Charting bullet points like, "Patient shared some very touching sentiments from her personal history regarding her grown son, including a few regrets that recur to her at times," are not likely to offend that patient if she reads them, and they add to the whole-person treatment towards which hospital culture is evolving.

The awe of witnessing the birth of one's own offspring and the saying goodbye at the time of death of either of you at any age, are both segments of the parenting arena, as well as all the giggles, little hurts and minor injuries, misunderstandings, and proud moments in between. What happens to the hearts of your children happens to you in some proportion. There has probably never been a day in which each of my children did not enter my mind several, often dozens, of times. Nobody seems to play the parenting role perfectly, without at least a few nagging regrets in old age. Yet hardly any parent would ever want to have missed that ride.

STORIES ABOUT GRANDPARENTING

Shortly after I took my first hospital chaplain job I met a woman in an isolation room who became quickly open about her life. She said, "I never learned to love from my parents," as she explained why. "I never learned to love from my husband," and she again explained. "I didn't love my children very well either, because I hadn't learned how yet. Where I learned to love was from my grandchildren. They were just so exuberant, free, and unbounded with their love." I asked if she was sad having taken so long to learn how to love. She said, "No. I'm just happy I did eventually learn before I die."

A retired grandpa fishes alone off the dock of his lake cabin at quiet dusk. His mind meanders from the ripples of his line to the sunset to his deceased wife of 43 years to the eagle fishing from a treetop across the bay. Somewhat abruptly the 16-year-old son of his only daughter trots down to show him the trophy he won this afternoon as part of the team competition in the Paavo Nurmi Marathon. The boy beams with pride, shares the highlights of the race, chatters of his father being proud, mentions some future hopes, and asks grandpa about his fishing. Almost as abruptly he mentions that he doesn't want to be late for supper, and jogs away with his quiet grin intact. Grandpa smiles, remembers his own athletic better moments, warms inside to the pride his daughter must feel, pictures his wife again, and quietly returns to his angling, his spirit buoyed by this brief but soulful visit.

Later life opens to this one entirely new arena to feed and challenge the spirit. Merely gazing upon the face of your own third generation offspring adds a whole new dimension to life. If a patient offers pictures, admire them.

On the other hand is the woman who most vividly remembers how as a little girl, when her grandfather would visit her family and greet her, he would stick his tongue into her mouth as he feigned kissing her. This relationship, like all spiritual arenas, can have its dark side.

STORIES ABOUT SIBLINGS

A "warrior dash" is a few miles of water, mud, and wild terrain through which venturous young people scramble at rapid pace for fun. My most treasured picture is one in which my three children stand together with their broad grins, covered with mud and arms around one another in glee after finishing a warrior dash in their 20s. Seeing your children vigorously enjoying one another stands with some of the best experiences in life.

Early sibling relationships are a mixed bag of joyful play, raucous mischief, pleasant memories, dogged loyalty, sad disappointment, stabbing hurt feelings, nagging worry, bitter frustration, and lingering regret. Later there may even be stubborn resentment-driven estrangement. Generally the longest relationships we ever have, sibling ties can make us proud. The one voice I could often hear over the crowd cheering for me in the small school gym where I did pretty well in basketball games was that of my sister June. Siblings can also make us deeply sad, as when at 23 I cried alone in the bathroom after June's wedding, realizing she would never be my sister in the same way again. They can hurt us deeply too, because they know some of our most intimate secrets and vulnerabilities. And they can surely embarrass and annoy us as I've done with my stupid behavior. When a patient mentions a brother or sister in any context, there may seem to be no spiritual need afoot. But a simple, genuinely curious response, followed by lingering, if you have the time, such as, "You have a sister?" may ignite a much longer story in which joys are celebrated and aches are aired.

The words of Samuel Butler in *Elementary Morality* still hold some truth however. "I believe that more unhappiness comes from this source (the family) than from any other—I mean...the attempt to prolong family connections unduly and to make people hang together artificially when they would never naturally do so" (Butler 1917, p.31). Beautiful as this pristine relationship can become, it often doesn't.

STORIES ABOUT FRIENDS

In unpublished doctoral research[2] comparing 35 of these spiritual arenas to one another from various perspectives, two stood out among all the rest in estimating which ones had fed respondents' human spirits the most throughout the eras of a lifetime. One of those top arenas was an interpersonal one—friendship, which some would call the crowning glory of all of living. In conversation that is deeper than social, almost nobody would remain silent to the topic of "fine friends we have had at various points in our lives." That conversation would also include stories of how badly some people who we thought were friends had eventually hurt us. The actual presence of true friends, whatever that term "true" may mean to a given person, is what we yearn for during our most difficult times. We generally can't put our finger on why a specific person, out of the wide variety of our acquaintances, became a solid friend. Half of friendship results simply from chance.

The other half, however, is responsibility. As the primary antidote to loneliness at various times in most lives, friendship magically makes some people special in our eyes. Some siblings become friends with one another and others never do. Some lovers become great friends and

---

2   Thesis by the author from 1988, entitled The Spirituality of the U.S. Spiritual Clinician, online at www.spiritualclinician.com/the-spirituality-of-us-pastoral-clinicians.html. It is a study of over 2000 chaplains, pastoral counselors and clinical pastoral educators regarding their experience of the spiritual arenas during the various eras of their lives.

most others eventually part. Some co-workers establish themselves as inexplicably giving us the "benefit of the doubt" as a first stance in whatever happens to us. Others at work seem to take the opposite attitude. The particular individuals who somehow become our friends, at least for certain periods of our lives, remain so only with our investment in them during their troubling times. The mystery of friendship feeds almost everyone. As Aristotle wrote, "Without friends no one would choose to live."[3] When a friend accompanies a person for hospitalization, or even visits her, there are stories there, and stories of betrayal by other former friends may also lurk.

STORIES ABOUT THE ELDERS

I was 16 when I got separated from the family hunting group with my uncle Frank. He was an uncomplicated factory worker, raising his three teenagers alone. We were looking for pheasants, moving slowly through a grove at the edge of a sod field with new light snow on the ground. We talked some, but he was a minimally verbal man of meager education and I an inward teenager. Abruptly he stopped, motioned for me to be quiet, handed me his shotgun and began to move slowly to his left in the sod field.

Startled, I held his double barrel and watched as he slowly approached a clump of sod, stopped, crouched, balanced his body, and then thrust his right hand under the sod. Up it came with a rabbit in it, caught with his bare hands. As we continued on, excitement leaked out of his voice and face as he shared how he and his six brothers used to hunt rabbits that way as boys, chasing the creatures on foot, pursuing them with the farm dog until the rabbit got tired or hid in a somewhat accessible spot. As he shared those bits of lore and personal history in such a dramatic moment, the respect I already had for him multiplied. I felt proud to be in that family and with the men. My sisters never got to see and hear neat stuff like that.

How we are regarded by the elders, the older men or women whose gaze we habitually feel, affects our developing young souls

---

3   Aristotle (1869), Book 8, Chapter 1, p.259.

more powerfully than we've attended to in recent decades. As Robert Bly asserts, "No boy comes to manhood without an older man who is interested in his soul."[4] The arena of the elders consists of *that aspect of life in which we interface with the older men and women during our formative years, incorporate their wisdom and ethos into our own person, and sort their identity from ours during early and middle adulthood.* The formative years can include at least the first three decades of life, and in some cases beyond.

Besides bolstering our identity and self-solidity, however, specific elders can also exploit or ignore us, leaving us few clues on how to be a man or woman with substance, identity, warmth, strength, and creativity. Spiritual caregivers ought not to ignore a patient's story about an elder—a coach, scout master, pastor, uncle, aunt, or neighbor, either in admiration or in disappointment, gratitude, or wounding. The latter may lead to a vitally important referral for abuse in childhood.

STORIES ABOUT TEACHERS AND MENTORS—AND STUDENTS

When the world was quite new to our daughter and she was in the midst of learning the power of saying words about it, I would sometimes take her down into our basement with me while I put wood into the furnace. At 18 months old she had already developed the habit of pointing with energetic enthusiasm and regal authority while saying, "Tzat?" which many parents will recognize as meaning, "What's that?" "The water heater," I'd say. "That's what makes the water so nice and warm for your bath." The garden hose, my bicycle reflector, the water pipes, a socket wrench, and countless other objects in that combination storehouse, woodshed, workshop, and pantry, were words for her to say and gain some fledgling understanding about. She was richly into the spiritual arena of *encountering the new* called learning.

Learning something new is an absolute delight. Despite the dismal attitudes that are common in public education, inspiration about what is new exhilarates the human spirit. Most of us carry stories about

---

4   Robert Bly, leader of the men's movement in the 1990s, in a lecture at Pacific Lutheran University, Tacoma, WA, February 13, 1991.

great teachers who "saw" us more fully, pastors who conveyed warmth at crucial moments, coaches who engaged our best hidden abilities, or mentors who helped us onto a new level of understanding, practice, and life. The entire endeavor of learning and developing as a person, including those who help us engage it successfully, constitutes a rich spiritual arena.

Stories about any of that—how one negotiated childhood classrooms and teachers of great or sour memory—are worth a hearing, even if they don't immediately seem relevant to a particular hospitalization. Remember that the word "doctor" essentially means "teacher."[5] Learning about a particular illness or condition that is now associated with your name needs to be a far more integral part of healthcare culture. Patient stories about great teachers may inspire a given physician or nurse to more creatively teach as a potentially rich aspect of their own care practice.

Still, I have a younger male relative who was molested by his teacher in the sixth-grade (age 11–12 years), throwing him into mass confusion for decades. A tragic story indeed, of the kind that hides deeply within until the right listening context emerges.

STORIES ABOUT GETTING HELP

Dressing a new infant requires you to do it all yourself, gently overcoming the wriggles. At about three months of age, however, you can begin to feel some cooperation from the little guy. He can help you help him. It may be years before he can dress himself, ask for help when he needs it, and stop asking for it when he really doesn't. But already at three months, he is introducing himself into the spiritual arena of help getting—*the slice of life in which a person elicits serious help when she needs it and cooperates with the help when it comes*. It includes the events in a lifetime in which a person learns to partner with a solid helper and use all the skills and attitudes it takes to make use of somebody's significant help for his own person—including counseling,

---

5   From the Latin docere "to show, teach, cause to know."

psychotherapy, consultation, going back home, and reaching out for what only an institution can provide.

Stories of the process of admission to the hospital, the life turn-around of addiction recovery, positive or dismal surgery results, and other tales about how one was pushed to the limit before seeking help can often be consolidated into a patient's personality by his recounting them at the precisely right time. That is because getting real help for oneself is a process that brushes against the essence of being human, our inherent vulnerability in the face of a fundamentally uncontrollable world. As an example, the transition from an addiction lifestyle to a recovery one stands as a powerfully spiritual experience, whether those words are ever used in the process or not. Getting real help for oneself changes a person fundamentally, placing us on a new life direction that includes getting help more easily the next time. Healthcare is full of helpers. And not all of them know how to get real help for themselves or even recognize when they need it.

STORIES ABOUT HELPING OTHERS

At 22 I went to Mexico to engage an idealistic mission of helping native priests in their work. Mostly what I gained was an appreciation of just how naïve and arrogant I was. Rainier Maria Rilke discovered that too, and wrote succinctly about just how difficult it is to really help somebody. In *Letters to a Young Poet* he said, "At bottom and particularly in the most important things, we are utterly alone, and for one person to be able to...help another, a lot must happen, a lot must go well, a whole constellation of things must come right...to succeed" (Rilke 2011 [1929], letter dated April 5, 1903).

David was a gregarious young priest serving a small Midwestern city when it was hit by an F4 tornado, devastating its structures and crippling its systems for weeks. Driven by youthful enthusiasm, Dave filled a borrowed truck with donated food on the second day and headed for the surrounding countryside. He spent the morning stopping at farms of families he had previously known to be less prosperous, only to be shocked at how quickly and solidly they rejected his help. He knew they needed the food he offered, yet they refused it immediately. They would simply not be open with him about their needs. Discouraged, Dave drove back to town and stopped at a little cafe where men tended to gather.

There he met with John, a simple-minded and outgoing fix-it man considered odd by many and harmless by everyone. Affectionately known as "Crazy John," he had an infectiously positive temperament that was often a day-brightener to townspeople. As Dave told his disappointing story, John took him outside. "Hey! Let's go try it again," he said as he got into the pickup. Puzzled, Dave again drove to the nearby farms, and this time he marveled at "Crazy John's" approach to people. The old man chatted, and listened to the stories of where the people were when the storm hit and what it did to their buildings. He responded to their tours of damaged structures, and even joked a bit. Before they drove off, he'd left the families with boxes of give-away food that Dave hadn't even gotten them to consider. Dave was taught that day by a truly humble, uneducated, and gifted helper.

Major religions have long fostered teaching about giving help to others. Charity in several forms is the substance of virtues taught in every church, synagogue and mosque. It is seldom, however, included in such teaching, that actual giving of help absolutely requires other genuine virtues such as humility, patience, joy, and peacefulness. Hospital staff are full of helpers who may not recognize that their work is deeply spiritual practice and that their attitude towards patients makes the difference between those sick and injured people feeling cared for on the one hand and being painfully ignored or even quietly insulted on the other.

Caregivers fairly frequently encounter an older patient who has taken care of people all her life only to subsist alone now, with nobody to care for her. In addiction recovery circles another common phenomenon is one who over-cares for an alcoholic for years while starving her own eroding life to a shambles. These unfortunates exemplify the pain side of the altruistic arena of helping others.

Personal spirituality: The diverse path towards self-treasuring

A Native American grandmother sought advice from a spiritual leader. "I'm raising my granddaughter, and I tell her every day that she is beautiful. But one day I forgot, and she reminded me. She had noticed her 'fat cheeks' and began to worry about her looks. I helped her fix her hair in a way that would distract from her cheeks. Did I do right?" "Appreciate her cheeks too," he replied. "For it is not her physical appearance that will win friends and lovers, but the light in her eyes born of a spirit delighted with herself and her world."

The path towards truly treasuring yourself is almost invariably rocky and never without personal disaster of some sort. The wars we wage between aspects of our own selves do not take place in the abstract, but in the contexts or themes we are calling arenas of personal spirituality. These come at us relentlessly, some daily, some in explosive intrusiveness, and some in messily progressive developmental patterns, all with the power to wound and yet all challenging us to greater levels of soulfulness with ourselves. Personal spirituality is this cluster of spiritual arenas in which a person encounters herself directly and repeatedly, with both her limitations and best gifts evolving ever more clearly in her view of herself.

STORIES ABOUT PHYSICAL SELF-CARE

The entire endeavor of healthcare exists for the sake of this one spiritual arena. Caring for the compromised body, when it has impinged on the human spirit with alarm, is the traditional overall mission of healthcare culture. Almost all patients have something significant happening in their arena of physical self-care, if for no other reason than the story of what got them hospitalized. The stories of admission and the reason for it often come first in patient disclosures. A serious spiritual caregiver can hardly avoid listening to the most obvious issues currently alive for this person, right now.

A major piece of caring for one's own human spirit is stewardship of the body that houses it. That is a far more complex job than it seems like it should be. Even when society discovers what is beneficial for the body we seem to resist acting accordingly. Obesity, smoking, excessive drinking, sedentary lifestyles, and sleep deprivation stand as solid examples. At times partnering with our bodies for the long-term benefit of our lives can actually seem impossible. But we are compelled to try. Physical self-care is *accepting the primary responsibility for care of your own body, getting consultative help for it when the need arises, and facing its limits when it breaks down.*

This arena presents spiritual struggles in two directions: tussles with ourselves in body maintenance and wrestling with higher powers when the body gets sick or injured or deteriorates. Stories of the latter are most common in healthcare, as patients begin to talk with spiritual caregivers by recounting what happened or what's next for their lives. Stories of neglect of one's own body are less common, but still are seen boldly in such regrets as those that characterize addiction lifestyles and the results of foolish adolescent risking.

EMOTIONAL SELF-CARE

Human emotions weave their way through all other spiritual arenas and in some form can be seen in every patient visit. Feelings always remain a quite mysterious aspect of human existence. They emerge from within our bodies with a life of their own from origins we variously recognize. They arise from the perceptions of our senses, relate themselves to our thinking, motivate our actions and color our memories. They provide most of the richness of life, including all of the joy. Emotional self-care is *the arena of life in which we become aware of our affective processes, intentionally care for them, and learn how and when to express them to feed our relationships and decide about them to direct our actions.*

Feelings live alongside logic to provide an entire other window on reality: *anger* to fuel our actions for improving situations for ourselves and others; *fear* to warn us of danger, either internal or external to ourselves; *affection* and *sadness* to tell us what we love and have loved;

hurt to show us what we truly value and signal our need for greater self-care; *guilt* and *shame* to self-evaluate our decisions and their effect on others; and *joy* to provide a cue on what to celebrate. A hundred nuances of each of those help us gain some bit of comprehension of the mystery perspective rather than the problem view on our surroundings.

Besides providing richness to life, all of these basic and universal emotions can burgeon into problems during hospitalization. When they do, or when they hide too deeply, they can spawn serious spiritual needs (see Chapter 3).

I was 29 when I discovered I'd been lonely most of my life. It was a great revelation to me, and an embarrassing one. I was successful as a clergyperson and capable of addressing some people's spiritual hungers. But when I identified the feeling of loneliness, and recognized it as what I'd felt most of the time as an adolescent and young adult, it was a humiliating acknowledgment and a promise of something different possible ahead. The first project of emotional self-care is to recognize what you're feeling life is telling you, and the second is to openly acknowledge it. These tasks rarely take place in isolation, but rather through a relationship with someone who cares about you enough to listen and tell you the truth. My CPE peers were that for me about loneliness (see the Epilogue). Hospitalization can be the occasion of that for some patients regarding their anger, their hurt, and even their fears.

WORK STORIES

My father was in his early 30s before he left the Iowa farm and married my mother. He tried several jobs and survived the Great Depression before settling in as foreman in a small dairy where he worked for 25 years. He hired whoever worked there for much of that time, and needed to decide which applicants would be able to do the job. He once told me, "You can always tell which ones grew up on a farm. They already know how to work." There is a "knowing how to work" that those who have become too self-absorbed, too wealth-preoccupied, too cynical, or too already-defeated-by-unemployment may never achieve.

Work feeds the human spirit and the right work feeds the soul. In one episode of the old TV series *Kung Fu*, the Chinese priest–protagonist enters a small Western town and is confronted by a local bigot.

> The man snarls, "What you lookin' for in this town Chinaman?"
>
> "Lookin' for work," says the itinerant priest.
>
> "Ain't nobody gonna pay you for nothin' around here Chinaman," spits the local.
>
> The priest surprises him with the response, "Not looking for pay. Looking for work."

Separating work from pay confounds us as members of a capitalistic society. But indeed work is its own spiritual arena and the joy of work is its own reward.

Talking about one's work can often reveal to the careful listener just how well that work fits or once fitted the worker. Segments of our society have forgotten the spiritual value of work itself, apart from money as one of its primary benefits. The Asian Kung Fu priest knows that he will feel better if he splits some wood or hoes some vegetables today than if he remains idle. The work one does for a living may not be the right work for him, but working itself is better than being idle for too long. The chronically unemployed suffer a double spiritual disadvantage: their bodies starve from poverty, their souls from lack of meaningful work. Women especially can become quickly and mostly quietly disenchanted with their work that is still often valued less highly than that of men.

Besides failure in finding truly enjoyable work, some primary directions that miss fulfillment in this arena are *preoccupation* with work and *disdain* for it. Preoccupation with work as an addiction short-circuits feelings by activity, and rationalizes the self-deceiving avoidance of intimacy with thoughts of it being "for the family." The reason for practicing the Sabbath in Hebrew tradition was to rest from work, rest your animals, and spend time nurturing and maintaining family ties. Like a mouthful of salt, living as a workaholic is too much of a good thing.

Disdain for work is equally deadening. The growth of "entitlement" in a society, by dependence-fostering government programs, exorbitant insurance or court settlements, or enormous lottery winnings tempt people to avoid the spirit-nurturing that comes with honest and fitting work. Hospitalization threatens this arena as a common worry of patients. Will they ever do their best work again?

STORIES ABOUT SEX AND SEXUALITY

Human sexuality constitutes a massive arena of its own, related to romance but separate too. Dealing with natural sexual urges in their unique and unpredictable rhythms continues to baffle us whether we are seriously engaging a romantic relationship or not. Feared, worshiped, disdained, and condemned by diverse political and religious groups throughout history, sex has been lavished with more attention than most any other aspect of human experience. Sometimes an intense and delightful upper, at other times a frustrating, baffling downer, it pesters people from adolescence to the creaky stages of aging, and remains as much a mystery from its first sparks to nearing the deathbed. As a spiritual arena, sexuality is *the lifelong pursuit of frequent enough intimate emotional connection and genital expression that promises to satisfy body, spirit, and soul.* And as M. Scott Peck (2010) once quipped on a widely distributed tape, "Even those who write the books about sex are mostly mystified by it in their own lives."

Sex is probably a unique experience for everyone but the common patterns that differentiate male penis-centered and testosterone-driven sexuality from women's emotional connection thirst and meaning/beauty search are well known. Songs like Bob Dylan and Ketch Secor's "Wagon Wheel" (Nettwerk 2004) and Dan Hill's "Sometimes When We Touch" (GRT TU 2750/20th Century Fox 2004) illustrate the pervasive male fantasy of a committed and enthusiastic partner dedicated to indulging him out of generous and understanding love. Female fantasies likely include far more emotional interaction and intimate interpersonal connection but also contain the element of a partner full of dedicated enthusiasm for her as a person and a carnal being. While much sexual interaction may be more love seeking than pure pleasure seeking, the aspect of indulging another as intertwined with being indulged simultaneously seems to be deeply embedded in the human soul (see Hilsman 2010).

Sexuality may not arise overtly very often in spiritual care conversations, but it is often there beneath. Concerns about loss of sexual potency with the progression of renal dialysis, certain medications, and some surgeries; pregnancy avoidance; abortion decisions and regrets; marriage or love life conflict; and societal attitudes towards one's sexual orientations that differ from the prevailing one are only a few that can be precipitated out by hospitalization.

In addition is the emergence of sexuality and sexual involvement in the helping relationship itself. Pastoral care students as well as those from other disciplines are often surprised and then secretive about their sexual or romantic attraction to specific patients. Finding the clear line between professional care and romantic involvement often takes crossing that line a bit in order for a fledgling caregiver to find it. When a caregiver gives indication to a patient or parishioner that he may be interested in a romantic or sexual relationship with that person, he has already crossed the ethical line. He needs immediate consultation, usually leading to the end of that relationship, or to change his job or social role. Hospitalized people need caregivers far more than they need new lovers. Yet because of the depth of their spiritual significance, the experience of processing such attractions in clinical supervision can be highly transforming for students and practitioners.

NESTING

My wife and I were sitting quietly at the kitchen table one evening after supper. The worn yellow linoleum had been loosening behind the refrigerator, and she drew my attention to it. I pulled up a corner of it to see how bad the old glue was, and casually commented that it looked like hardwood underneath. A moment later there appeared in her eyes the glint of mischievous inspiration that I've come to know means things probably won't be the same for a while. We spent all free time for the next three weeks removing three layers of glue and refinishing that hardwood floor and those in all three upstairs bedrooms. The moment had catalyzed a semi-major event in the arena of nesting.

The nesting arena is *the segment of life in which energy is expended in the arrangement, maintenance, and enjoyment of your own living space*. It includes on the dark side the tragedies of home invasion, homelessness, and that house burning down. In clinical settings it is the latter three that are most likely to arise in conversation or otherwise present themselves for care.

Everyone has a history of nesting. The project of arranging your own living space ranges from claiming part of a room shared with a sibling in childhood to fighting for your privacy in the nursing home at 80. When you first realize you have some freedom to influence the way it looks and feels around your sleeping space at home, you're beginning to be affected by the nesting arena. And there is frequently at least one tragic event in changes of one's abode. My wife's uncle was a tough, crotchety curmudgeon when she helped him move to a nursing home from the house he had lived in with his wife for over 40 years. As Nancy carried the last box from the house she looked back and saw him actually kissing the house goodbye.

MATERIALITY: STORIES ABOUT MONEY AND OWNERSHIP

I remember as a five-year-old once seeing my father sitting on the couch with his head in his hands, unusually pensive. My older sisters were there, and we were all somewhat mystified about what was happening in Dad. We asked, and he replied that he was figuring out how to get enough money for a down payment on a better house. How the three of us kids decided together I don't remember, but sensing strain in our father, we emerged a few minutes later, offering him our piggy banks, with whatever paltry change they contained. We must have thought we could really help. It is the effect our money has on our hearts and those close to us that affects our spirits and souls, for enjoyment, distress, or resentment. As a spiritual arena, materiality is the name given to *the ways one relates to material value*, which in a capitalistic society means mostly to money and what it can buy.

Money indeed does feed the human spirit. Dad referred to how "that money is just burning a hole in your pocket, isn't it?" And an old Yiddish proverb states, "With money in your pocket you are wise and you are handsome. And you sing well too." Shopping enlivens most women, and robust bottom lines do something similar to men. One of the seven deadly sins in the medieval Catholic tradition pointed to the spiritual peril of being encased in greed so firmly that relationships and other values suffer.

When patients talk about money it generally isn't because they have too much and don't know what to do with it. They are worried about paying for their care, or otherwise not having enough for what they and their families need. The topic of money can feel like a minefield to a caregiver because manipulation is so easy and prevalent around money, and because there may be little one can do except refer to a social worker. But often, sharing money concerns with a trusted somebody is enough.

HUMAN DEVELOPMENT AND AGING

At 35 I was consulting a psychotherapist, largely about my foolishness in relationships with women during the 18 months following my resignation from the priesthood. I'd felt embarrassed to even disclose details about it, and whined a bit about being 35 and acting so crazy. He quietly commented, "Everybody has to have adolescence."

My perspective changed. My adolescence was late. So what? It began to seem much more OK to be somewhat stupid about dating in middle age. So what if my adolescence was in my 30s. I learned something that day that I'd partially learned previously with a master's degree in human development. Development just is. It is more important to get with your current point in its progress than to evaluate and even judge yourself about being behind in the process.

Time relentlessly moves on, and it shows—in our bodies, our attitudes, our knowledge, and sometimes in our experiential wisdom. While the pace and quality of our development can be influenced a bit by our intentional action, the movement of time is beyond us.

The spiritual arena of developmental aging is made up of *the natural tasks, unfolding joys and inevitable limitations of decline we meet in progressing through the life cycle*. A framework of development casts light on almost any patient in terms of the challenges and obstacles that show themselves during the various eras of a human lifetime. But any hint of moralizing regarding what stage a person finds himself in at any age is likely to be counterproductive in helping that person meet the messes inherent in that stage.

The classic radiant exuberance shining from the face of a child who has just taken her first steps from dad to mom signals a very early expression of spirit stemming from the developmental aging arena. Simple and unsteady, they are monumental in her life. The wisdom of an aging man who has cared for people, made contributions to society, and embraced his approaching end manifests that spirit too. The patient's age in whatever stage of life, and his attitude about it, matter.

Transcendent spirituality: The awe and dread of transcendence

The third axis includes eight arenas in which we encounter the "beyond," or transcendence, either more directly or organizationally in religion. In healthcare settings in which caregiver eyes frequently meet the strained faces of pained people, there is a tacit awareness that all healing involves an element that transcends humanity itself. Experience has taught reflective IDT members that nobody knows in many cases why one person heals and a similar one doesn't. Sometimes that is unsettling. Sometimes it is awesome—or awful.

When a child or young mother patient either improves unexpectedly or deteriorates inexplicably; or a grotesquely injured accident victim dies screaming for help that cannot come; or a critical teenage girl lingers on and on for days without improvement, the emotional experience digs into caregivers' souls. A few staff members cry and hug. Others isolate themselves, secretly stunned by unsettling sensations in the chest or the pit of the stomach. For many people that profound experience has no name. History has called it awe.

Awe can neither be controlled nor explained. Just short of overwhelming, awe is essentially a mildly debilitating mixture of penetrating emotions—quietly stunning fear, vague sadness, gnawing inadequacy and a curious sense of unworthiness. Experiences such as standing a few inches from a deadly precipice, watching a baby being born, and observing somebody finally die, all evoke that brief, vivid awareness that, "There is obviously something far bigger than me, bigger than all of us, going on here." The magnificently awesome and the dreadfully awful similarly command our respect.

Awe punctuates our typically vague awareness of a power far beyond the human that is constantly operative right in front of us and even sometimes palpable upon reflection. In experiences of awe, transcendence is made obvious. Like the rain to a child, a shower that cannot be stopped by anybody, they are signals of the "beyond" that sometimes become just short of tangible. They bear the very meaning of spirituality within them, the vividly uncontrollable that has always fueled human efforts to cope with and enjoy an inscrutable world. Some patient stories emerge from every vivid experience of awe.

MAJOR LOSS

Intensive care staff met in a conundrum over a woman being kept alive beyond usefulness of any care to her condition. Her son, her only relative, was adamant that she not be abandoned by the healthcare system. His stolidly immovable attitude repelled them all, in its intense, submerged hostility and tireless intractability. A chaplain happened to visit the young man on a drop-in visit, mostly unaware of the situation. In the course of their conversation, he discovered that the young man's father had died three weeks before. As the young man verbally processed the experience of finding out about his dad's death without having said any goodbye, and as he talked about their long-time contentious relationship, he reminisced with tears about the few good times he could remember about his dad, and the pervasive yearning for more of him during most of his young life. This was his last parent. The dying mother presaged his being orphaned. He was grieving actively and effectively for the first time. The change that took place in him seemed almost miraculous to the staff, as he immediately began to collaborate with them about his mother's care.

The universal theme of major loss constitutes some of our most vivid and obvious experience of transcendence. Seeing somebody dead that you love, or dying and not being able to stop it, can convince us that there are powers much higher than ourselves as clearly as anything else. If there weren't such powers we wouldn't be losing what or whom we're losing. The ache inside takes us over for a time. We can't stop that either. Humanity has spent hundreds of years evolving ways of dealing with the incomparable complex of emotions we now call grieving. The hundreds of books on the process published since C.S. Lewis's *A Grief Observed* (1961) have not removed the mystery from that mess of feelings and ways of coping with the loss of somebody or something treasured.

Hospital experience commonly brings to the surface losses that have been poorly grieved or even ignored (see Chapter 4). And even those losses we've grieved quite thoroughly rise up, mostly unexpectedly in warm, sad emotions that can beckon forth further reminiscing and tears.

Being a patient for a time can precipitate further integration of past major losses into our personalities, consolidating and expanding on what those losses have taught us and the rich ways in which the people we have lost have deepened us. Our lives are made up of many people and things that we have and had only for a time. The uneven process of transforming the pain of loss into the gratefulness of what we have received stands as a most fundamental spiritual achievement that tends to happen primarily in dialogue.

STORIES ABOUT ONE'S MORTALITY

As a young priest I was serving two tiny farm towns east and west of Highway 65, which runs north and south of Rockwell, Iowa. One extremely foggy Sunday morning I was driving from Swaledale to

Cartersville, moving a bit too fast, probably thinking about how to improve my sermon for the second mass. I suddenly caught sight of the stop sign on Highway 65 going by and I shuddered to realize I hadn't even slowed down. Almost simultaneously a car driving south passed in front of me and immediately another going north, passed in back. As I realized I had been split seconds from being slammed by one or the other, or both, I knew I had come as close to death as I had ever been. My mortality whacked me as hard as either of those cars could have. It was not my first emotional brush with mortality but certainly the most dramatically memorable.

A few stories about near death experiences lurk in the corners of most everyone's minds. As John Donne (1923, p.98) reminded us so pointedly, in words first published in 1624, "And therefore, never send to know for whom the bell tolls; It tolls for thee." During hospitalization, brief proximity to many people who are dying or could be dying, frequently brings home the reality of ultimate mortality to patients, however quietly. The entire experience for many people edges them closer to emotionally facing the logical fact of their eventual dying. It peeks through habitual denial if only for a few brief moments. Such thoughts are typically shared very selectively. When they are, however, they are likely to prepare us just a bit more for actually facing the fact of death when it comes.

STORIES ABOUT NATURE

When my sister's oldest son was reeling from a recent divorce in his 20s, I asked his mother Joyce where he was. She said, "He's headed for the cabin up north. Nature's where the healing is." It is likely that all spirituality emerged first from human encounters with the beauty and peril of the natural world. Even today, it is a rare individual who is not moved, at times deeply, when standing by the ocean, walking in a blizzard, or witnessing a hurricane. At the same time there is great therapeutic power in nature. The writings of Sigurd Olson articulate this spiritual aspect of the wilderness as well as those of anyone else (Olson 1946): "Wilderness to the people of America is a spiritual necessity, an antidote to the high pressure of modern life, a means of regaining serenity and equilibrium."

The natural world has been taking care of and threatening us humans like a mother for a very long time. We've relied on her, taken her for granted, used and abused her, built to shield ourselves from her, been calmed, inspired, and healed by her, and we continue to be awed by her. We are fed so much by nature that we bring little bits of her into our houses as pets and plants. The time is approaching, like with most mothers who live long enough, for us to need to take over care for her, treat her better, protect her, be cognizant of her limitations, and replenish her the best we can in times and places of extra need.

It is likely that all spirituality originated with humans regarding the natural world, including both its beauty and its devastation. The oldest human artifacts appear to be fertility figures, depicting wonder at procreation, one of those arena transections where the natural world, interpersonal mystery, and personal spirituality dramatically meet. When calamities come from the natural world she is often seen as an instrument of a punishing god, blaming people for her not being what somebody thinks she should be. But nature has always combined grand beauty with ferocious violence. It is in that combination that nature, and all spiritual arenas, boldly manifest the mystery with which we constantly live. Patients' stories about nature, climate, weather, beauty, hunting, environmental action, and whatever else illustrates the mysteries of nature, spring from awe at either the glory or the tragedy. Honor them.

PERSONAL DEITY

One pivotal point in the evolution of human efforts to meet transcendence functionally was some bright humans beginning to see that inscrutable and overwhelming power as personal. For a long time the Hebrews resisted putting a name on that experience of awe. That would reduce the power of the experience. But if logic could have been applied to that transformation it might have sounded something like this: "The most advanced creatures we know are us, people. Whatever that is that we sense in the sun, the moon, birth, death, and natural disasters must be at least as advanced as us. So we can talk to it. We ought to." It would be thousands of years before the immediate, lighthearted conversations with God of Tevye the dairyman in Shalom Aleichem's story on which the musical *Fiddler on the Roof* was based, but prayer had been invented.

Almost everyone prays, at least reflexively, when severe trouble looms over them. It doesn't take much, just a few authentically urgent words. But it can be difficult to determine upon reflection whether or not you're only talking to yourself. Far different is the depth of earnest pleading, "storming heaven" it's been called, when one desperately wants something big for oneself or for someone dear. That kind of prayer doesn't necessarily get you what you requested but it does seem to change the person praying. Prayer can also be calming, enhancing one's perspective, creating a direction. If nothing else, it locates the source of power outside oneself to some degree, taking pressure off oneself in some situations. It shares the burden with some power greater than oneself, injecting a feeling of being less alone in the world. Praying together earnestly with somebody else can be even more reassuring. Praying with people prescriptively, that is, focusing a prayer concretely on the needs felt by the patient and named previously in conversation, is an essential skill of spiritual caregivers.

Any mention of God, Allah, or even "the man upstairs," can be an occasion of deft entry into how a patient images transcendence. Even proclaimed atheists have an image of what it is they don't believe in. The wide variety of ways people image transcendence, or even preach about it with excessive certainty, probably serve them well. It helps them cope. Of course none of us really know much at all about transcendent power. When we speak of transcendence as personal, we put aside knowledge for a bit and enter into the world of belief.

The troubling side of a personal transcendence belief is still seen frequently in hospital situations in patients who feel guilty and being punished by their condition for doing what they believe they shouldn't do or for neglecting what they should have done. Intense, existential guilt and fear of eternal retribution by an angry God still stalks a number of ill, disabled or dying people. Hearing the stories of those regrets and responding with genuine care remains a common spiritual caregiver role (see Chapter 4).

RELIGION

My father knew little about theology beyond the Catholic catechism. He dropped out of 11th grade (age 16–17 years) just before the Great Depression to take over the farm for his mom and the other ten living kids of his increasingly dysfunctional father. But Dad was quietly faithful about Catholic practice. I never heard him preach about it to his children nor anybody else. But in his last years I asked him about his daily habit after retirement of walking the few blocks to the local church for morning mass. He simply said, "I'll probably always do that."

Almost all ethnic cultures include a religious component. As cultures were forming, ways of relating with the powers obviously active all around were apparently a necessary element. Over the eons of history, the efforts of the world's great religious leaders to improve humankind's spirit care have brought useful concepts and practices to billions of people over the centuries. A confusing few of those beliefs and practices are visible on any hospital service. Apart from the theological skirmishes and divisions in each of the world's great religions, most people get compelled by some of the classical, traditional religious ways of seeing the world. They mostly ignore what makes no sense to them in the teaching of the religion of either their heritage or of their choosing. And they strive to act in accord with what feeds their souls and what makes sense to them to guide their behavior.

During hospitalization, however, some particular questions tend to come to the fore in people's minds. Instances of feeling manipulated, fooled, coerced, or downright abused by religious leaders also may arise in the pensiveness of hospital time spent in bed. Complex as the religion arena is at this point in history, it stands as a major spiritual arena and likely will for ages to come. Humanity cannot easily wipe away centuries of development of those efforts at seeking conscious contact with positive transcendence. Hospitalization naturally rekindles patchy positive effects that religion has had on almost all of us. Five specific religious needs that arise frequently in hospital care are described in Chapter 3.

THE ARTS

Whether in creating beauty or merely enjoying it, the arts affect everyone, in different ways and on different levels. Everyone is compelled by at least one type of music, for example, and a few exceptional individuals actually compose symphonies. Stories depicted in theater once stirred people around primitive fires as well as they did last night on Broadway. Great novels have inspired people, taught them, and enriched them now for centuries. Human efforts to illustrate for other people the magnificence and tragedy of life in poetry, theater, song, and artifacts makes art an arena of the human spirit that cannot be ignored by a sincere listener. The question, "Did you see such and such a movie and that scene where so and so did this or that?" captures how art helps us express those emotions and attitudes for which we cannot find adequate words ourselves.

The five-year-old who enthusiastically presents her mishmash of crayon color for parental appreciation hazards the same risk as the would-be novelist waiting for a publisher's response to his first submission. While art is rarely a key arena for hospitalized people to express themselves, still there are times when a certain piece of literature, tear-jerking song, or movie scene makes the difference between a patient feeling deeply understood or left alone with an issue that continues to vex him. Art pieces are points of contact between souls. Leil Leibowitz (2014, Preface) put it this way, "You feel the same at a Cohen concert that you do at a church or a synagogue, a feeling that...the words and tunes...represent the best efforts we humans can make to capture the mysteries that surround us..." What intuitive care is needed to choose the art on hospital walls? And who will hear the story of the musician whose injury will prevent him from ever playing again?

COSMIC HARMONY

A colleague of mine—formerly a nun, a peace activist, a chemistry teacher, and a professional chaplain—saw a transformation of her basic spirituality later in her life. The Hubbell telescope photos manifesting anew the stunning magnitude and majestic beauty of the universe in its astounding complexity shook her into questioning her lifelong image of God. She doffed her 60 plus years of active Catholicism for practice of Unitarian Universalism, which allowed her to remain theist without seeing the Deity as a person. Mystified by that rather unusual change for a woman already steeped in science to master's degree level, I asked her why. She could only say that the universe appeared to be so real in the pictures that the idea of a God in heaven slipped away from her. She could still pray but her prayers were less intimate now. Was that conversion a step ahead in spiritual development or a step back?

I had long since resigned myself to the mystery of that question, its inability to ever be answered clearly. The universe's evolutionary process leaves little room for a personal God. Yet our human makeup needs communication with whatever it is that is obviously so far beyond us. Both ways of seeing the universe are valid. Fortunately I had found in a modern physics class in 1962 that one can mathematically prove that light is a wave and equally certainly prove that it is streams of quanta. Our ways of seeing the transcendent similarly can be mutually exclusive of one another and yet both be true. So evolutionists and scientists can pray in gratefulness and theologians can follow the logic of an ever-expanding physical world, seeking metaphorical meanings of heaven and an afterlife that don't make literal scientific sense.

Isn't our best truth that nobody can say anything about a transcendent being for sure? It's a matter of belief, not philosophy or proof. In the evolution of religion, the transformation from fearing and respecting obvious transcendence as an impersonal, sometimes brutal cosmic power, into relating to transcendence as a benevolent and magnanimous personal being was not universal. Buddhists, for example, and many scientists would rather seek harmony with transcendent reality as a system of physical forces than see the highest power as personal. They still treat transcendence with great respect and even reverence. Speaking intimately with those forces as if they were father or sister is generally not a part of that style of spirituality. Christians, Muslims, and Jews on the other hand, more likely believe that verbal communication with the Beyond is possible and even easy. Like Tevye in *Fiddler on the Roof*, such conversation they believe, is a hallmark of the spiritual life. Any mention of God by a hospitalized person prompts a spiritual caregiver to heighten her alertness for religious needs and issues (see Chapter 4). Helping a Buddhist or an atheist spiritually is a different but not necessarily a less important task. Humanist concepts help in either case.

Communal spirituality: Belonging and gatherings of all kinds

We humans are basically quite communal beings. That patient you're caring for grew up in a family community, was probably educated in classes, exercised and competed on teams, worked collaboratively, joined clubs and associations, and lived in neighborhoods. We humans fashion cities, create nations, contribute to societies and connect with one another across the planet in internet groups of many kinds. We do that because gathering in groups of people with whom we have something in common buoys our human spirit, helps fend off isolation and loneliness, inspires our purposes, and feeds our souls. Care-full listening to patients includes alertness to what communities or groups with which a given person connects with authentic energy and how those communal relationships are going at this particular time. There are at least eight kinds of communities that comprise the fourth cluster of spiritual arenas, which we can call communal spirituality.

FAMILY OF ORIGIN STORIES
The field of addictions treatment spurred almost folksy concepts on the tendencies of dysfunctional family siblings to form patterns based on their place in the sibship.[6] As is commonly known now, in response to

---

6   The consecutive order of siblings in a family.

an alcoholic parent, oldest siblings tend to become super responsible, second ones to be distracting with mischief, and so on. For example, when Sheila begins to share about how she took responsibility for the care of her three younger siblings when she was only nine years old herself, it raises a stark question about her role in that family. Very likely she was the family hero, at least for a time. She is likely to be super-responsible, painfully so, unconsciously taking on some of the duties of several of the people around her. Freddy, who says he did time in juvenile detention three times before he was 18 is just as likely to be living the pattern of a family scapegoat, who learned early that being good had no payoff for him and to get attention it would have to be through negative behavior that was aggravating to those around him. Getting insight into these patterns won't necessarily stop them, but if the situation shows patient readiness, that insight may give these two patients more options about how to make serious decisions in the future.

Every family consists of an absolutely unique context that has as much influence on shaping sons and daughters as anything else in their subsequent lives. The roles of the different family members can be seen in reflection on the question, "What was your role in the family when all members were assembled?" Group theorists and family therapists describe how we all tend to recreate our family of origin in groups in which we are involved. Spiritual caregivers functioning in hospitals have a role in eliciting patient awareness of the influence of their family of origin on their development. The stories of their childhood and youth convey isolated pieces of that influence, ranging from heart-warming memories to ghastly tales of abuse and neglect.

ETHNIC HERITAGE STORIES
When I went to Mexico in my early 20s, in naïve hopes of helping out native priests, I discovered that people could be living in *pueblecitos* that geographically were surprisingly close to one another while speaking totally different language dialects. In Huehuetla Hidalgo, where I was, the native dialect was Ketchwa. The mountain on which my friend

was living was close enough for me to see it, but the language there seemed to have no relationship to Ketchwa at all. Apparently, when those languages were developing, members of the two communities never came in personal contact with one another.

There developed eventually on this planet over 6000 ethnic cultures, well over a thousand with their own unique languages. Cultures are so diverse with unique foods, marriage customs, religious practices, and traditions of dress because they all evolved completely separated from one another over periods of thousands of years. Only in the past few hundred years have domesticated animals, wheels, ships, airplanes, and now TV, cell phones, and the internet brought us face to face with these very different ways of being in the world. We're forced to face that our ways are not necessarily better than anyone else's, though we have long believed that they are.

Eventually, in the continued evolution of a cooperative world community, some of those cultures may be lost. And even today, meeting hospital patients, ethnic and cultural diversity remain huge as we continue to be called to care spiritually for diverse peoples in the public institutions of this pluralistic society. Honoring and learning from ethnic differences will remain a major spiritual arena for a long time to come. Every one of us harbors biases of various levels of unconscious suspicion, annoyance, and assumed entitlement. As many have said, diversity of ethnic backgrounds enriches us all. But the negative side of this arena is, of course, still highly visible in racist policies, superior attitudes, those ubiquitous unconscious biases, violent altercations, and even wars. Patient stories of being misunderstood, excluded, overlooked, or marginalized may be difficult to elicit from people of oppressed minorities, but if they can be heard, they make a caregiver an island in a still stormy sea. And as caregivers we need to continue unmasking our own subtle fears of differences. We've come a long way in my lifetime alone.

NEIGHBOR AND NEIGHBORHOOD STORIES

My wife and I had lived in our 42-home neighborhood for about ten years before an even longer-time resident became active in facilitating our collective preparation for disasters. Len began to invest in convincing the rest of us to establish a program in which we would eventually have a plan of what to do in any disaster that might traumatize our city and in particular our housing division. Having a plan gives you something definite to do when things go sideways. You can move quickly without much discernment. We developed committees, each with a specific mission, including construction evaluation, first responding, medical/nursing care, communication, and even care of the pets in any emergency. After those few months of organizing, the neighborhood felt much closer, even though about 40 percent of the residents did not participate. We'd had a few summer evening block parties before that project but the ones we had after it felt a lot more cohesive.

A neighborhood is essentially a set of relationships based on proximity of residence. The primary affinity that may draw neighbors together is simply that they live nearer to one another than to other people. The relationships that develop beyond that are sparked by other similarities noticed by seeing one another and conversing by happenstance. There is potential for actually becoming a core cohesive unit made up of some neighbors, to which others remain peripheral but still belong. A microcosm of the human race, each neighborhood offers potential for real community on the one hand and violent or devious exploitation on the other. If we could watch a neighborhood in its constantly changing dynamics, we would probably see an inherent energy gradually forming itself into a rich reliance of neighbors on one another and a constant jousting with forces that tend to defeat that unifying process.

When you know a little bit about a patient's city and its various neighborhoods you can sometimes understand that person just a bit better and demonstrate that affinity with knowledgeable listening responses.

GENDER GROUP STORIES

The process by which a gay or lesbian person "comes out" is essentially a series of shared stories that are almost never told to straight people. Finding one's way into membership of a group of similarly gendered people can be circuitous and lonely. There is a clear connection between adolescent suicide and sexual orientation.[7] Tortuous as it can be, and extended in time, it becomes a project of joining, finding one person who can lead you into communal belonging. One colleague of mine knew he was gay before he was eight years old. Another says she didn't recognize her sexual orientation until her 47th year, her 20th as a mother. There is no definite timetable. But the more the stories are told, the more confidence seems to be garnered by the storyteller.

One lesbian CPE student of mine confronted her entire peer group at mid-unit with her observation that none of them had included any verbatim presentations involving a gay person as patient or family member. She wondered how they managed to unconsciously avoid that topic. She helped the group of us recognize some of the communication habits by which we assume heterosexuality in people and thereby discourage patient disclosures that would need to reveal sexual orientation. "So, are you married?" for example, and "Does your husband come to visit you?" While these questions can be answered by a person who is comfortably out, they most likely won't be by many out of politeness, muting further possible disclosures. This arena emphasizes a more general point about the caregiver's own stories and the unconscious biases that affect and sometimes deter any significant openness of patient conversations.

WORK GROUP

Relationships with co-workers may not strike caregivers as spiritual territory. But the effect they have on our human spirits can be enormous.

---

7   See, for example, S.T. Russell and K. Joyner (2001) "Adolescent sexual orientation and suicide risk: evidence from a national study." *American Journal of Public Health 91*, 8, 1276–1281. For more information, see American Association of Suicidology (www.suicidology.org) and The Suicide Prevention Resource Center (www.sprc.org).

Many of us actually spend more time with co-workers than with our families, and co-workers have a unique opportunity to join together in a common endeavor—accomplishing whatever the basic work is and sharing in the satisfaction that it generates. Work enthusiasm comes from working together on something we care about, and with people, at least some of whom we actually care about.

People with whom we work can also get on our nerves and deplete our spirits since we may not be able to escape, put distance between them and ourselves without quitting a job we like or need. The necessary collaboration the workplace requires can become so excruciatingly frustrating that we actually resist going to work for long periods of time. Any stories that put a light in a patient's eyes when she talks, or a shadow over her face, are spiritual stories and they need a listen.

PEER GROUPS

A Central American in his 30s was admitted to the psychiatric department of a large urban medical center for suicidal ideation. A chaplain quickly ascertained that he was gay and deathly afraid of his rigid Catholic parents ever finding that out. It would jeopardize their social acceptance back in his home country. It was that bind that had catalyzed his depression into what precipitated his hospitalization. He requested that the Protestant chaplain call for a Catholic priest to see him, refusing to say why. In conversing with him the chaplain concluded that what this patient needed was to learn how to make adult decisions for himself, and stand firm against his parents. He'd decided not to refer the young man to one of the staff priests available, even knowing that one of the staff priests was gay too. Could the patient not have benefited from a Catholic religious leader who was presumably understanding of the patient's family bind, to advise him? Didn't she neglect to note that the priest and the patient were peers—both Catholic, both gay, and both in excruciating conflict with religious regulations that hadn't yet evolved to be functional for their natural spiritual situation? He needed a peer group more than a challenge to take charge of his own life in a way that was likely impossible for him at the time.

Sometime after discharge the man did act on and complete his suicide plans. Peer groups can be crucial for a person's next stage of human development. The most effective treatment for addiction is carried out in small groups of similarly defeated peers, not one-on-one counseling alone. One middle-aged alcoholic patient in his first treatment for addiction put the power of peer groups this way: "I'd probably die for some of these people in here that I've only known three weeks. But my drinkin' buddies I've known for decades? I can't even get them to bring me a pair of socks!"

Similarly, the best chaplain training programs feature groups of five or six members to optimize the small group dynamics peer feedback intended for student benefit. And the most significant changes in physician practice behavior are seen in educational programs in which they are facilitated to engage personally with one another in small groups (Berkhof et al. 2001). The stark identification with one another that characterizes facilitated peer groups generates both validating feedback and challenging critique that are incredibly powerful for personal and interpersonal change. Whether they are peers in gender, sexual orientation, age, school grade, diagnosis, or life problems, it is similarity in some major aspect of life, some palpable affinity that pulls people together in one of the most powerful change modalities there is—the peer group. Reflective peer group members invariably notice an almost mystical energy both inside themselves and among them, in an uncanny cohesion that can develop in their group simply through shared experience in talking seriously about themselves.

The destructive aspect of peer culture is seen in the negative peer pressure that can lead members to make foolish, communally deviant, and self-defeating decisions as is commonly seen in high school clique bullying, and violent gangs.

FAITH GROUPS

Faith groups subsist as organized religious communities of people holding similar official convictions and regular practices. For more than a billion Muslims around the world, for example, finding a place to kneel, bow, and pray alone or together five times a day remains a challenge, especially in the workplace, when traveling or when hospitalized. For them Ramadan is a "month of blessing" every year, marked by prayer, fasting, and charity. Once in a lifetime a pilgrimage to Mecca in Iran is a profoundly moving event.

The Roman collar of traditional Catholic priesthood dress still carries a powerful religious significance to millions of Catholics, despite pedophile scandals that embittered so many churchgoers in the early 2000s. Sacraments retain great meaning for some Catholics and that fervor gets multiplied by illness and injury. Morality decisions can nearly paralyze a staunch Catholic during medical ethics challenges such as unwanted pregnancies and increasingly futile care. Dogma may be decreasing in influence over the planet, but it is still alive and powerful in many ways.

Proponents of religions that feature gathering regularly with other members as a prominent way to keep their faith alive can feel especially misunderstood or ignored when their religious life position is not recognized by anyone around them in their hospital. In addition, over centuries, some faith groups have painstakingly fashioned solid moral positions that have become rigidly encased in regulation and passionate, non-reflective adherence. Common spiritual binds such zeal causes in hospital situations include the complete avoidance of blood transfusions by Jehovah's Witnesses at all cost and the committed covering of women's faces in public by some Muslim sects. But religious conflicts in health care can be far more complex and hidden in people who are situationally intimidated by alien cultures and technological starkness. Teasing out such needs takes empathic persistence, which itself requires a special sensitivity and a caregiver's quiet, dedicated relational time.

A "modern world" view easily dismisses religious piety as obsolete. And religious need is admittedly a tiny fraction of the spiritual needs in hospitals. But religion's importance in a fair segment of the population's lives and research studies finding its value will not let a humanistic spiritual caregiver ignore it. In fact, religious people will probably always be only narrowly understood by any caregiver who has no religious belief herself, and no practice that is vital to her.

NATION

Standing on that hill in Lexington, Massachusetts, where in 1776 about 77 farmers with muskets faced the approach of hundreds of the finest soldiers in the world, brought tears to my eyes in 2014. Though those incredibly courageous men and boys didn't withstand the volleys very long, the experience of standing in their place tweaked a nationalist pride that still lives within me. I have long preferred a total world view to a nationalistic one. But like many who visit Lexington and Concord where the combat phase of the American Revolution began, I can still exude patriotism, feeling the courage and grit of those first civilians who stood, knowing they could now be executed as traitors. The ragtag packs of Americans with an intense desire for the cohesiveness it takes to be a country felt a power within them, an excitement, a burly resolve that we call rugged patriotism. It remains a major force among peoples of the world, which results in speeches, parades, and celebrations every year in many countries. It also still propels thousands to their deaths in war and revolution.

Military veterans, especially those who have seen combat, harbor stories of their military service, only rarely finding an acceptable context in which to give them verbal expression. When a veteran shifts into storytelling mode, it is generally after a breakthrough conversation with similarly wounded peers at some point in his or her past.[8] A caregiver with the time, interest and skill at close listening, helps heal just a bit, the wounds of armed conflict, gradually freeing that teller

---

8   About 1.8 million of the 22 million US military veterans are women (www. pewsocialtrends.org/files/2011/12/women-in-the-military.pdf).

of horrible stories that desperately need an appreciative and grateful response. The breakthrough conversation in which that complex of stories begins to blurt out can then be followed by connecting them to facilitated peer groups where the sharing can flow at least a little more freely.

HUMAN COMMUNITY

A common Amish question in their communal decision making reflects that group's dedication to simplicity: "What will this do to our community?" It has been suggested that such a deliberation is also a great one for the people of the world. There are two kinds of people: those who sincerely ponder this question, and those so preoccupied with other interests that they don't consider it in their business operations, religious leadership, philosophical perspectives, or theological understandings. But the global community that is relentlessly and unevenly forming still includes a wide swath of those who have not yet joined the global community movement. For the latter group, humanitarian efforts still appear to be nothing more than political maneuverings, personal image enhancements, or financial advantages in tax benefits. A genuine commitment to improve the living conditions of the world community has not yet appeared on their radar screens as worth personal investment.

The evolution of humanity proceeds anyway. The nature of evolution has always been full of what seems to us as enormous waste. As it continues to unfold, it encounters myriad setbacks and pushes on regardless. It can reasonably be suspected that a major segment of any hospital staff now is motivated by empathy for the human spirit and making a contribution to the race as a whole. It is no longer only a few religious groups such as the Amish, devout Buddhists, liberal Catholics and Social-Gospel Protestants, who are overcoming sectarian religious squabbles, ethnic differences, and historical resentments. The human community is coming together, albeit way more slowly than humanitarians and many "ordinary people" would like.

A segment of most every society has been twisted in the winds of intense conflict during this evolution of a global community. Combat veterans, torture victims, sex trade abductees, and child laborers all exemplify the millions of painfully wasted lives as the cultures on this planet negotiate their conflicts towards eventual global collaboration. Members of all of those groups find their way into hospitals and have stories to tell. When they do, it becomes clear that their tearful narratives have been invariably held tightly within them in the vacuum of words that such brutal treatment inflicts on the human spirit. Any bit of healing that can take place in them begins with somebody able and willing to listen, teasing out story after story in preparation for engaging effective treatments, some of which are only now being created.

As a spiritual caregiver listens with concentration to the stories in these 35 arenas, her ear is alert to what current *spiritual needs* are being disclosed in any of them. Such needs are of course, innumerable. But direction can be found in a framework of needs that are seen repeatedly among hospitalized people. Such a framework in common terms allows a caregiver to quickly identify spiritual needs, focus descriptions of the unique needs of this particular person's spirit, and more easily organize them for IDT members. Twenty-two such needs, along with suggested goals of care, are described in the next chapter.

3

Content

I thirst.

CRIED OUT BY JESUS WHILE DYING[1]

It is what happens within the primary spiritual arenas that constitutes spiritual needs, the content of spiritual care, and recording it in the medical record. Dr. Gregory Fricchione, Director of the Benson-Henry Institute for Mind Body Medicine at Massachusetts General Hospital, has developed a general theory of illness and injury centered on the ways in which they tend to isolate human beings who then need help from professionals for reattachment strategies (Fricchione 2011). Sickness, disability, wounds, chronic conditions, and major loss all set us apart at least temporarily from everybody else. The primary

---

1   Bible, John 19.28. It can be argued that this near death statement was at least partially
     metaphorical, referring to the way in which this influential spiritual leader had
     apparently yearned all of his public life for the betterment of people's treatment of one
     another, especially at the most difficult times of life.

function of all physicians, and by extension all helpers, he summarizes, is to assist people to establish or re-establish connections.[2] Hearing the stories of that process of isolation—its loneliness, pressures, fears, and inspirations for transformation—is a major component of whatever it is that helps patients move towards healing.

The ancient story of Job powerfully illustrates this separation as he is depicted as being personally detached from everyone in his life by loss and illness. At those times in life when things radically change forever, it initially seems that nobody at all actually understands what it is like to be us. We walk that lonesome valley alone, at least for a time. All forms of genuine care have at least one thing in common. They serve to stimulate people to either remake connections with other people or develop new ones that transform them. Hospitals are places where almost everyone who is seriously challenged by their reasons for being there is challenged as well to let themselves be remade, giving rise to the possibility of connecting differently to the world—potentially better than they were doing before, albeit now with more compromised physical health. That is the nature of healing. In one of the two endings of the Book of Job, he goes away with greatly expanded perspectives of what the world is really like.

Spiritual needs have been conceptualized in various ways over the centuries, though not by that name. Eternal salvation, freedom from guilt, inspiration for increased hope, serenity, and feeling close to a positive transcendence are a few such historical renditions of spiritual needs posited by religions. For our purposes, however, we use the term "spiritual need" as applied to the limited area of the experience of hospitalization. Rather than philosophical correctness or conceptual exactness, we focus on identifying needs commonly felt by hospitalized people and recognized frequently by experienced spiritual caregivers. And rather than focus research data on observations of what chaplains

---

2   See Fricchione, 2011, pp.458–459: "The mystery of this separation-attachment process is most profoundly felt at the bedside where the stakes are highest. The physician-scientist must engage in a practical consilience of inductions if he is to attempt to cure as well as care for his patient by finding attachment solutions to his patient's separation challenges simultaneously on multiple levels."

do, our intent here is to describe needs as seen in patients. Healthcare is comprehensively arranged by patient needs. Identifying *spiritual* needs is congruent with that tradition.

Clearly defining goals to meet spiritual needs in humanist terms is relatively new. It follows the lead of palliative care practitioners who have adopted the term "goals of care" for figuring out how to prescriptively address the unique desires and hopes of suffering people in creative ways. Spiritual caregivers working in those specialized services have been challenged to not only contribute to the program goals for a given patient, but also to add their own spiritual goals that fit with the program's medical goals for that person. That push has been a healthy one for chaplains involved. The process of reflecting on and writing spiritual care goals helps to give spiritual caregivers direction in participating with IDTs in focusing on identified issues of patients rather than being content with the common practice of assuming that a genuinely personal caring relationship helps virtually all people. The practice of defining specific goals challenges the broadly accepted pastoral care assumptions that listening, encouraging, supporting, advising, guiding, and praying with people in the midst of life's difficulties actually bolsters them against their predicaments.

Those common assumptions have been proven over and over again informally through observation in the professional lives of chaplains. Still, as often-repeated and almost ritualized written goals, they can become inane justifications for reticence or inability to engage patients and their issues more deeply. Supportive care, for example, a staple among established chaplains, fails miserably when it is the only approach applied to most addicted patients, undiagnosed mentally ill patients, those with simmering medical ethics issues, family conflict situations, and almost any other specialty spiritual need. Yet that supportive care is generally a solid place to start in initiating the helping relationship. It helps establish rapport. It serves as a platform on which to base other, more specific goals of care.

In order to promote creative development of spiritual caregiving, we can distinguish between *general* goals of spiritual care based on

90 years of history of clinical chaplaincy, and *specific* goals of caring for any given patient. Specific goals can only be fashioned in the immediate context of encountering a given person. And the infinite array of goals that may be best for any given patient can become a bit more manageable when organized in the context of spiritual needs commonly seen in hospital care. First, however, here is a summary of the general goals as intuited from chaplain experience and the clinical ministry literature.

General goals of spiritual care

Any clinician interested in improving her spiritual care of patients within her own helping discipline can learn a great deal from the history of clinical chaplaincy. Generally, goals for spiritual care can be described based on the history of the clinical ministry movement beginning during the 1920s (Hemenway 1996). Listening to patients in the new ways of eliciting their own core concerns discovered by the depth psychologists of the late 19th and early 20th centuries radically changed chaplaincy and set it on a different path from previous styles of practice. The new style of chaplain pursued goals, largely unspoken and unrecorded, centered on establishing a depth of rapport with patients rather than the previous best practices of advisory, supportive, and ritualized religious care of as many people as possible. Clinical pastoral education as the educational initiator of hospital ministry concentrated on the inner world of the chaplain in preparation for forays into the field of the inner worlds of patients. From the history of the resulting clinical ministry movement we can identify at least the following general goals of care for most all patients.

I. *To connect emotionally—to make meaningful human connection and establish rapport adequate enough for the caregiver to receive stories and disclosures about spiritual needs from the patient's point of view.* The assumption here is that what is of greatest importance to people is what they feel most vividly and deeply about at any given time. CPE students are guided and prodded to listen carefully for hints at what a given patient is feeling and for clues as to how to engage them about their basic concerns. Much of the clinical training of chaplains involves developing this competence.

2. *To convey empathy that clearly shows a person that the caregiver understands at least one significant aspect of that person in some depth regarding how it is to be her at this time in her life.* Once a caregiver perceives or intuits an indication of significant concern in a patient's emotion and disclosure, next he finds a way to show that person that he understands the depth of the matter, at least to a minimal degree. The themes of learning the intricate art of conveying genuine empathy pervaded basic pastoral care education before the recent emphasis on research to measure its effectiveness.

3. *To communicate the genuine warmth of acceptance, verbally and non-verbally, to all people as they present themselves, regardless of such potentially dividing considerations as faith group history, sexual identity, ethnic culture, moral situation, language, or appearance.* Radical acceptance,[3] made up of conveyed empathy and personal warmth, cannot always be portrayed with integrity and effectiveness. It may need to be intentionally generated by reflection on a patient's situation. Universality here is a basic characteristic of a humanistic approach that authentically celebrates diversity in people with a reasonable degree of humility based on awareness of one's own historical and residual biases. Even a hint of moralizing sabotages this goal.

4. *To promote trust of the caregiver(s) and the caregiving system.* As a component of depth of rapport, there is no substitute for a significant capacity to help people feel the caregiver's integrity, an almost palpable belief that this person operates her practice with consistent dedication to helping whoever she can that

---

3   The term "unconditional positive regard," as made popular by Carl Rogers, best illustrates radical personal acceptance (see, for example, Carl Rogers (1965) *Client-Centered Therapy*. Boston: Houghton Mifflin).

is in some kind of need. If a patient develops interpersonal trust in some member of an IDT then that relationship can be a point of promoting trust of the team in general, despite some members who may not demonstrate that degree of interest in the intricately interpersonal aspect of life or the personal integration that is required in order to linger there.

5. *To enhance spirituality, and support, empower, and build on the patient's own current best ways of bolstering her own human spirit.* It has long been recognized in the clinical ministry movement that crises like hospitalization are very seldom opportunities to teach or "correct" theology or change people's spiritual convictions. While there may occur needs that cry out for guidance and new understandings, for the most part the project of spiritual care is to build on patients' own personal strengths and spiritual resources, whether those are well established already or built recently on new felt needs.

6. *To challenge behavior, and gently, firmly, prescriptively, and incisively confront perspectives that may be defeating or sabotaging this person's human spirit.* CPE groups feature learning skills of confronting, or drawing attention to, important incongruences in a colleague's disclosures, affect, behavior and stories, without alienating them with moralizing advice or patronizing contention. Many spiritual caregivers still need further development of this skill however, in their patient care practices. Without some level of skill in the confronting art it is impossible to contribute to teams who are addressing patient conditions such as alcoholism, mental illness, and self-neglect.

Fashioning specific goals of spiritual care

Specific goals of spiritual care are brief descriptions of what caregivers think they can do and plan to do to address aspects of the patient's pain, discomfort, and deficiencies in their sense of purpose or meaning. The task of spiritual caregivers on an IDT can now be seen as essentially to contribute to fashioning and pursuing goals of care. This role has two parts. The first is documenting how spiritual care can participate in the clinical team's joint goals of care. The second is identifying any additional care goals from a spiritual perspective. Often, relevant needs emerge from the unique rapport facilitated by the spiritual care listening of tuning in to people's inner world without asking them too many direct questions. As a caregiver listens in this way, there is then a need to organize what the patient discloses in terms that convey to IDTs the tensions and binds felt by this particular person right now.

Some electronic medical record (EMR) systems require documentation of goals of care as necessary for access to making further entries into the chart. That insistence challenges spiritual caregivers to think carefully about their work before they write, and translate their care into the medical record through the lens of the goals of care language. To be relevant, goals of care are based on needs of patients as seen by the caregiver. Spiritual caregiver goals need to be in some way congruent with those goals identified by the IDT.

Experience helps in the process of identifying spiritual needs. As clinical chaplains have engaged patients over the past 90 years, patterns of need have emerged that can be helpful in identifying goals for any given patient. There is no possibility of creating an exhaustive list, nor is there a need to. Spiritual needs are probably even more complex than, and as numerous as, medical needs. Developing a useable framework of needs that experience has shown are common can facilitate the fashioning of unique goals of care for most patients. Those goals can be described in bullet points, paragraphs, or stories in the medical record. The following is a framework of needs, and their possible related goals of care are offered as a basis from which to function as an organizationally and personally integrated spiritual caregiver, and for some to study the results with future research.

These 22 needs are divided into four clusters based on four questions that play around the mind of the spiritual caregiver. The questions are not intended to ever, or at least commonly, be asked of patients.

Skilled personal listeners remain wary of too many direct questions, of over-focusing conversations on what the caregiver wants to know rather than what is actually concerning the patient and family. Still, a few general internal questions guiding the caregiver's listening help to focus on what is actually needed by this patient that is relevant to her overall care.

The four organizing questions used here are:

1. *What does this patient need from me emotionally right now?* The resulting cluster or axis of needs is divided into seven emotional support needs with their accompanying suggested goals of care.

2. *What has this person lost, historically, recently or anticipatorily, that continues to cause significant and sometimes distressing warm and sad memories?* Five common, almost universal major loss needs are identified in this cluster.

3. *How does this person uniquely maintain her own human spirit?* Five common religious and spiritual practice needs make up this cluster.

4. *What does this person need that is beyond what I may be able to provide?* Five referral needs make up this axis.

Descriptions of these 22 needs and their suggested goals of care are not intended to be cookbook menus of how to respond to them when recognized. They are rather named here to promote understanding by a caregiver that then invites sensitive, empathic, and conversational attitudes within which a patient can gain perspective and perhaps improve any ways the patient has been coping with, avoiding, or addressing the needs herself. Figure 3.1 illustrates these needs and how they relate to the task of assessing a given patient.

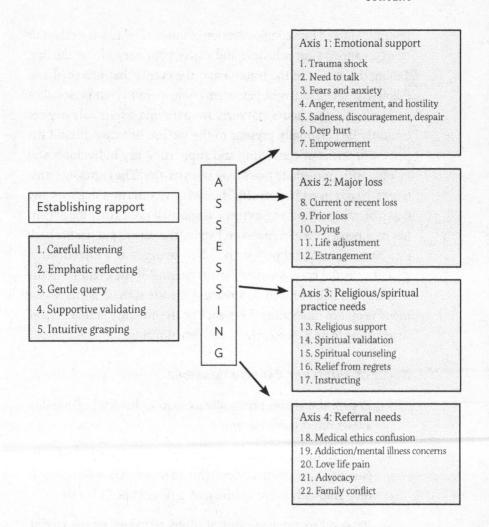

Figure 3.1 Spiritual needs framework

Axis 1: Seven emotional support needs

1. TRAUMA SHOCK NEEDS

Sometimes the human spirit becomes overwhelmed. To some degree it becomes at least temporarily disabled. While almost all reasons for hospitalization could be called crises in the lives of the patients, trauma experience stands alone in its severity and lifelong personal imprint. Marked by a conglomeration of intense feelings, it steals your energy, cancels your schedule and places your very life on the line. Telling the stories of the trauma and the events that preceded and followed it becomes a new, persistent component to your personality.

During the first hours that surround a trauma, a spiritual caregiver can only be personally present to the victim. But care *around* the person in terms of contacting and supporting key individuals and helping with immediate tasks may be extensive. The regressive state (see "7. Needs in empowerment" below) of victims overshadows any depth of interpersonal engagement as spiritual need. After the patient has regained a level of composure, helping the person put her life back into some meaningful perspective often emerges as a fundamental goal of spiritual care. Another person hearing of the event from the victim's own point of view in a relaxed, private context is crucial for many people in integrating the event into the life story of that person. Attempting to do so too early can be revictimizing.

GOALS OF SPIRITUAL CARE TO CONSIDER

- Engage the victim personally as soon as his level of stability allows direct conversation.

- Thoroughly hear the account of the crisis event from the patient's own point of view with all of its life implications as they gradually occur to him over a relaxed period of time.

- Respond to any mentions of ultimate values by the victim, with further listening and clarifying interest.

- Offer shared prayer when it appears that the victim is a religious person or otherwise may feel supported by a religious ritual or engagement of a positive transcendence.

- Facilitate the victim's planning for the immediate future in a prescriptive and timely manner.

2. NEED TO TALK/EXPRESS

A great percentage of people benefit from verbally processing situations and events serious enough to interrupt the managing flow of everyday anxieties with which we all live. In other words, most of us like to talk about what is seriously concerning us, and somehow forming words and sentences about it helps. While the felt need for such energetic talk varies considerably among patients, care communicated by personal attention from a knowledgeable listener with a calm demeanor invites spontaneous sharing of the many concerns fostered by hospitalization or unrelated ones brought with the patient upon admission. There is an enduring need for somebody on a team to listen personally to virtually any given patient in order for that person to feel emotionally connected and valued amidst the alien culture of healthcare. *It is most often through this care that other spiritual needs are identified.* Spiritual needs typically emerge quickly in a personal listening conversation, but always lie partially hidden by such phenomena as Spartan stridency, embarrassment, reticent personality styles, or unfamiliarity with finding words to represent one's experiences.

When a person has clearly shown a need to verbally process, it can be assumed that care has been conveyed and in a sense a new vulnerability has been born. That person now naturally expects someone in her surroundings to understand her better and listen personally again and again as she negotiates the concerns of her situation. This expectation may not be met in the current healthcare culture, but it is a form of care for a person to know that some understanding ears are available on the staff.

GOALS OF SPIRITUAL CARE TO CONSIDER

- Linger long enough to help the person relax into broad intimate disclosure regarding [any needs that occur to her] for further information...

- Identify further needs based on patient disclosures in the rapport.

- Consider return visit and/or referral to other caregivers, to address specific identified issues either during hospitalization or after discharge.

3. NEED TO REDUCE FEAR AND ANXIETY

Fear may be the most common spiritual need associated with hospital care. We all get at least a little queasy when we or somebody we love gets admitted. Sometimes that tiny fear burgeons to reticence and even refusal to agree to treatment regimens or surgery. But mostly that apprehension pokes along in our gut near the threshold of our awareness, emerging only episodically for some further knowledge, assurance, comfort, or support.

This bodily inclination to flee, hide, or frantically defend in order to avoid harm rises to some degree with any threat to wellbeing that is perceived as serious. Fear and anxiety, both seeking action and relief, are practically distinguished from one another by the clarity of what precipitates the emotional impression of alarm. Anxiety floats more diffuse and unidentifiable. The cause for fear tends to be more obvious. We are generally aware of what we fear. Anxiety seems more pervasive. Most patients experience some level of one or the other. When that level rises beyond merely uncomfortable to mildly disabling, the human spirit is exhibiting a need that can benefit from spiritual care. Chronic anxiety, as noted above, can significantly complicate medical treatment in ways that can often be mitigated, though never "fixed" by professional care, including medication. By our definition, psychiatric and psychological care do qualify as spiritual care. Skilled spiritual caregivers can address lower levels of fear and anxiety through quiet presence, careful listening for exploration of the sensations, teaching meditation or other perspective enhancing practices, prescriptively addressing the Deity to share the fright, i.e. prayer, and by referral to other professionals who would otherwise be unaware of the need.

GOALS OF SPIRITUAL CARE TO CONSIDER

- Reassure, without overstating hope unrealistically.

- Explore possibilities for facilitating the personal presence or support of established relationships of trust.

- Consider shared prayer, even regularly, as an experience of the presence of positive transcendence.

- Provide education/instruction—many of us relax a bit with specific knowledge we can trust. General understanding can be offered to some degree by a spiritual care person, or refer for more specific instruction from clinicians.

- Consider referral or suggestion of assessment for anxiety medication in situations of severity.

4. NEED TO MANAGE OR HEAL ANGER, RESENTMENT AND HOSTILITY

From a practical point of view, the human spirit of virtually every hospitalized person is being challenged, stretched, and even insulted by medical need and even some of its care. Being sick at least annoys us. The natural result of that is a measure of submerged annoyance, sometimes burgeoning to aggravation and occasionally even hostility. "Old anger," the energy of which seems to come from a patient's history more than the current situation, is signaled by edginess, verbal sniping, personally challenging tones of voice, criticizing of one's care and one's caregivers, threatening behavior, and sometimes violence.

Resentments from the past, of anything from severe historical injustices, such as having had a nasty or neglectful father, to a seemingly unfair romantic "dumping" can lodge themselves into our personalities and persistently affect our prevailing attitude. They do not respond well to religious efforts to heal them like "forgive your enemies." First, they hide. They perk along inside us unawares. Only when they are pointed out by some trusted observer do we make the connection of our current negative tones with the past hurt. In recovery programs for addiction resentments become a vital focus of interpersonal work because they sabotage sobriety or at least the joy of relationships in what is colloquially called a "dry drunk" nasty attitude. But they also inhabit the inner recesses of many less addicted folks.

When we become hospitalized, resentments exacerbate the natural levels of discontent that emerge from being disabled by a condition we simply don't like. Spanning a continuum from situational annoyance to violent rage, anger can cover over other emotions, especially hurt and fear. But the popular quip that "anger is a cover for fear" is clearly not always true. Anger is most of all a sensate message to our consciousness in big letters, that there is something going on that we don't like. Expression of the reason can be quieting, but in some people it only escalates the rage. It can best be seen first as a natural way of facing unwanted affronts to our comfort, i.e. *hurt* itself, and then *fear* of being hurt again, both crying out to be heard.

We naturally want to avoid those times in life that so radically slice into our inherent vulnerability. Some religious practice and theological thought are intended to prepare us for it. The meaning of the word Islam, for example, is "submission." Muslims are taught to submit to Allah five times a day, which can be seen in humanistic terms as preparation for the unpredictable worst times of life. Some standard Catholic practices—prayer before submitting to sleep, grateful sentiments expressed before eating, and the offertory of the mass that urges people to give all they have over to God—can likewise be seen as submitting to a supreme being that somehow loves every one of us in the midst of life's tragedies, as preparation for meeting the worst, both "now and at the hour of our death."[4] The Evangelical Christian practice of asking and allowing Jesus to enter into one's heart similarly requires a surrender of your own ego in order to obtain a measure of forgiveness, peace, and guidance for the unpredictably challenging events of your life.

---

4   See the Hail Mary, a common Catholic prayer repeated 53 times when praying the rosary.

In clinical settings, what is often encountered in patients, however, are bits and pieces of this teaching and practice that never deeply affected the patients and family members involved. Some caregivers tend, consciously or not, to avoid angry patients as much as possible. But what might observably angry behavior mean? What is causing it? What has hurt this person enough to let angry responses take over his behavior? As a component of most peoples' grief, each incident of anger deserves a closer look. It also needs caution. Acting out anger can be dangerous.

What should be the goals of care for meeting an angry patient or loved one? Who will assess the degree of anger in a patient, on the continuum between violent rages on the one hand and mere nagging annoyance on the other? A caregiver seriously interested in caring for the human spirit of even potentially unstable patients would be well advised to develop some level of these skills. There are other disciplines far more appropriate to meet overt anger in the hospital, such as security personnel and mental health professionals. But on a lesser acute level, almost all hospitalized people are experiencing more than one thing they don't like. Some level of anger lurks beneath the politeness of most patients, indicating at least a minor and possibly major disturbance of the human spirit. Responding to most of those levels of anger is a responsibility shared by all caregivers, including spiritual ones.

GOALS OF SPIRITUAL CARE TO CONSIDER

- Listen further for the possible emergence of the roots of the anger, in old hurtful events or recent ones, particularly immediately before or during this hospitalization.

- Avoid expecting the angry one to know too clearly and to be able to quickly communicate the reasons for the anger. Those reasons may be mostly unconscious.

- Elicit disclosure of major hurts that have prompted or exacerbated the anger, old or new.

- After quietly conveyed empathy, consider a story about functional use of anger from the caregiver's experience and memory.

- Address specific hurts disclosed, and consider offering to be an advocate for any current ones, within realistic limits of the caregiver's ability and availability.

- Consider inquiring about the patient's personal and/or religious history regarding injustice.

The following mini-case is, as all case notes presented here, constructed with imagination and a pasting together of reflections from memory of chaplain students in verbatim reports circulated to their clinical pastoral education (CPE) peer supervisory group for feedback and critique. CPE interns and residents are required to record their observations, emotions, impressions, reflections, and self-evaluations as part of the verbatim reports they regularly process in a peer group. In some programs they also submit the chart note they wrote to represent the care provided. The three sections of the reports below are the introduction to the verbatim, the analysis of the interaction after the visit, and the chart note written by the student. The suggested chart note improvements at the end are provided by this book's author.

ANGER ABOUT DISPARAGEMENT

Introduction

After visiting patients for pre-surgery at 6:30 a.m., and starting to chart on them, I had a referral from the previous night. There was a chart note in her file that stated: Patient is a 47-year-old single female who was admitted at night with bipolar disorder. She has been disruptive and was raising her voice at the nurses. More information also revealed that the patient lived alone and had no family in the immediate area. There was also a referral to have a chaplain visit her, which was written by the head nurse. There was no information on how the patient ended up at this hospital.

I immediately felt some angst from previous encounters with people who had bipolar episodes, and some of them were not at all pleasant. All I could think about was, "What am I getting myself into?" As I started to head towards the elevator, I felt a sense of peace come over me, and realized that I was trusting in myself again, and I needed to be thinking about the patient. "OK," I said to myself, "Let's put this in perspective," and off I went.

When I got to the floor, one of the nurses asked me if I was here to see the patient in 2-West. I said yes, and she looked relieved. I said, "I heard it has been a long night." She said, "Yes, it has. Please go visit her." As I entered the room, it appeared very dark; there was just a little light on beside the bed, there was no sound at all in the room, no TV, no music. The female patient was lying on her right side and had several blankets on; she was alone. She was expressionless.

Analysis

The patient had asked for a chaplain to visit her. She appeared to be a little confused on how she ended up at the hospital. She seemed depressed and wanted someone to comfort her and just be there. She defiantly had an agenda for the chaplain, and that was to read the Sermon on the Mount (the Beatitudes) and the fruits of the spirit. I think she wanted to know that she was accepted in God's eyes regardless of how others viewed her. During our conversation I think she eventually started to understand that she was loved and accepted by Him. I think that she actually knew why she was in the hospital, but refused to accept it or didn't know how to. She did not talk about family members at all.

Chart note

Patient is a 47-year-old female who was distraught and became very anxious during our visit, to the point of screaming. She had requested a visit from the spiritual care team. Upon my arrival and a quick visit with the nursing staff, I was informed that the patient had arrived the previous night by herself and was very disruptive. At first during our visit she was very despondent but after asking me to read a specific verse in the Bible, she became quite vocal and agitated. She mentioned that her friends all thought that she was not being righteous, and she was outraged by these comments. After a prayer and another verse of scripture she settled down and wanted to get some rest. I intend to stop back by to visit the patient again to see if we can find out some more about her friends, and where her family is.

Suggested improvements

Patient is a 47-year-old woman who requested to see a chaplain after being admitted alone the night before and being disruptive with the nursing staff. Nothing was known by staff about any family members. She initially seemed despondent and asked me to read specific sections of the Bible, about Christian virtues. She became vocal and angry when talking about a group of friends who were vigorously judging her as "not righteous."

- *Goal*: Assist patient to improve her self-worth. Chaplain listened to her, assured her of her worth in God's eyes, and read more from the Bible after she calmed down.

- *Goal*: Explore conflict with friends. As patient's medication is adjusted I intend to follow up with her, hoping for a calm conversation about the events with her friends, naming the hurt under the anger. I also hope to add further perspective to her view of "righteousness" and her value to God, and explore with her, her life, isolation, and possibly her family situation and history.

5. NEED TO SHARE SADNESS, DISCOURAGEMENT, DESPAIR

Sadness is the feeling of diminished enthusiasm for life, an unpleasant mood of discouragement, or impression that you've been enduring something for a while and are now "fed up" with it. In clinical practice it spans a continuum from missing a pet in a long hospitalization, to discouragement with the droning fatigue of a prolonged dialysis regimen, to quietly planning suicide. Rarely does it respond much to cheery encouragement, and it is exacerbated by feeling alone and that nobody anywhere really understands your situation.

Muted emotions are not the sole responsibility of psychologists, social workers, psychiatrists, and other psychotherapists. What is depressed in depression is the human spirit. Caregivers interested in human spirit care may not be qualified to diagnose clinical depression. But addressing sadness and discouragement are part of their role. They might want to invest in continually learning how to refer patients to other professionals for evaluation of what could be depression on the serious end of the discouragement continuum.

Discouragement, literally loss of courage, was a key element of assessment for Alfred Adler, an early Freud student and later competitor. He would frequently hold as a diagnostic question the internal query, "What has discouraged this person?" Whether a caregiver uses the same words or not, that can be a caring question for any fellow human being to ask herself. Similarly, a simple observation such as, "You seem sad," when the interest it conveys is genuine, may be a fine first step in responding to low affect. A clinically depressed person will not usually answer those questions usefully, but a sad or discouraged person is likely to feel like she's found a friend. Sadness can be seen as a continuum, from a Monday mood, to considering termination of dialysis, to suicidal depression.

GOAL OF SPIRITUAL CARE TO BE CONSIDERED

- Explore the reason for the sadness, perhaps starting with a recent and then long-term history of major losses or hurts from mistreatment.

Finding the reason is not likely to heal the sadness but it may initiate a process of grieving that eventually will diminish, and on occasion even transform it. Eliciting the sharing of sad emotions and repetitive memories that habitually remain internal may in itself restart an unfinished grieving process that needs more sharing in order to proceed (see "Axis 2: Five major loss needs" below). Open reminiscing about the good times with a lost one, even by divorce, can often be facilitated to the palpable relief of the sad one. The bad times are easier to remember and share. Sharing the good times brings tears.

END OF THE TRAIL?

Introduction

I visited the patient in his room on the 5th floor last Saturday just before noon. He is a 77-year-old rancher who lives about 40 miles south of Farmerville and over 150 miles from Metrocity. He recently came to Metrocity to receive treatment for esophageal cancer over at Stotz Cancer Center. When I met him, he was sitting in his room in a recliner. His hospital gown was pulled aside, revealing the gastrostomy tube coming out of his abdomen area. He is a large man, with a chunky body, a full face and a head of thinning gray hair. As I entered, he looked sad and stressed.

His wife was sitting on a chair just inside the door. She was wearing a western-style shirt, blue jeans and boots. She has short, wavy, mostly silver hair and a weathered face. As I entered, she looked stern, almost angry. Later, I realized after talking to the patient and his wife that she was worn out and frustrated.

The patient and his wife were in need of encouragement and peace. They had come up against a brick wall: nothing seemed to be going right; they were pushed to the edge. And now they wanted help; and they needed to know that they could ask God for help, that God loves and cares about them, even though, as the patient put it, they had not been going to church.

Analysis

The patient was at a low point in his stay so far at County. He had come in for a procedure that was to make official, make visible, what the esophageal cancer had already mostly accomplished: taking away the patient's ability to enjoy eating food by mouth. And now the device installed in that procedure was not working, and he was not able to even be fed by a tube inserted directly into his stomach. This, on top of being away from his ranch and his cattle...his life, really...plus being in the midst of radiation treatments for his cancer, which is likely not comfortable...and he was really in a mess. He was sad and so frustrated he looked to be on the verge of tears. His source of support is his wife who is trying to tend to the ranch, which is hours away, and her husband, whose condition is getting more complex. And it turned out that she too was on the verge of tears. I was struck by just how alone the patient and his wife seem to be. I wondered whether they had children or siblings somewhere and, if so, were they available to help? I wondered about this patient's self-identification as a Methodist and yet the sense that he has felt separated from a faith community for a long time. Is that by choice or because he lives in such a remote area that he has no access to any Methodist or similar congregations?

Initially, based on the patient's wife's demeanor, I sensed that I was walking into hostile territory. She was clearly upset, frustrated and even angry about something. She was even a bit scary, for she seemed so masculine and tough. But almost the first words out of her mouth were that they needed prayer. However, I didn't just pray right then. I got them talking about what was happening and then after all that, we prayed. Should I have prayed with them right then, after her statement? Possibly. But I took her statement to be one of exasperation, not a literal request for prayer right then and there. Yet I knew that bottom-line prayer was what they wanted. The patient seemed weary and frustrated, but I was not put off by his appearance, like I was with his wife. I found myself once again wanting resolution to their problems. I had trouble envisioning my role as simply to care for them in this moment. I wanted to do more.

Chart note

Patient is a 77-year-old male rancher from out beyond Metrocity. Patient has been receiving treatment for esophageal cancer at Stotz Cancer Center and was admitted here for gastrostomy tube placement. Just before my visit, nursing staff apparently attempted to feed him through the feeding tube, but the tube appeared clogged. Patient stated that the nursing staff were still working on it. He appeared upset and frustrated about the situation; both he and his wife seemed on the verge of tears. These are the difficulties they are facing:

- They have a ranch four hours away that needs tending at least every couple of days; Patient's wife has been going back and forth from there to here; she appears worn out.

- Patient's cancer treatment has been stressful; they have accommodation this week at some place called Valleyway but it seemed they were uncertain what will happen after this week.

- Patient and his wife do not appear to have a good support system; there is no close family in the area, and they depend on neighbors to watch out for the ranch, which has been threatened by fire already this year.

Suggested improvements

Patient is a 77-year-old rancher who is beleaguered by the encroachment of his cancer and its implications for him and his wife. Sadness pervades them as these tough homesteaders face the emerging impossibility of maintaining their quite isolated ranch as age and chronic illness sap their energy. Patient's wife immediately asked for prayer, as they remain without church support in their area. Patient's wife has been traveling the four hours (each way) back and forth to maintain the ranch every two days as his treatment here seems to them relentless. The chaplain listened extensively and prayed with the couple as both of them showed tears.

- *Goal*: Gently address the limits of the future of ranching. I hope to follow up with them and confer with the social worker regarding any family or other sources of support available, and consider the timely advisability of approaching them about their considering selling the ranch. They may be already experiencing anticipatory grief.

---

6. NEED FOR UNDERSTANDING AND HEALING OF PERSONAL HURT

Gus is 6 foot 3 (190.5cm) and weighs 225 pounds (102kg), but he looks small when he talks about his childhood. "I remember a long time in 3rd grade (age 8–9 years) when it was the worst. I was a skinny little kid, and I got into a thing where everybody picked on me. No matter what I did I'd get beat up. Every night after school at least two or three of 'em would chase me. I remember running out of school as fast as I could to get to the firehouse. If I could get there I'd shut and lock the door and wait for them to go away. But I knew I couldn't stay there forever. I couldn't sleep there. So after an hour or so I'd open the door and try to get the rest of the way home. Usually they were waiting somewhere and I'd get beat up anyway. It seems like it was always bad but that time in the 3rd grade was the worst. Nobody would ever help me."

The vulnerable sensations evoked by hospitalization can bring back memories of major hurt from past events. Hurt as a feeling easily gets neglected by most of us, as we favor being seen as angry or even fearful. But hurt lies at the base of both anger and fear. What we fear is being hurt—again. What makes us angry is that somebody has stepped on the toes of something we value highly. Both involve hurt that is unintentionally shielded from view. Disclosing hurt actually makes us more vulnerable. Somebody can laugh as a response, which intensifies the hurt. Unconsciously, both anger and fear seem better choices to feel than naked hurt. Seldom does anybody actually recognize our hurt. When they do, and gently say so, it can be a balm to the soul.

In the marked vulnerability of hospitalization, hurt can be caused easily by aspects of the healthcare culture itself. The effect of hearing curt phrases, impatient tones, or feeling neglected by a caregiver can result in stinging feelings that resemble the heart pain of a romantic breakup. One such event can quietly destroy patient satisfaction and even trend a person's attitude towards lawsuit. In addition, there exist a surprising percentage of people who live with the interior deep wounding of past trauma, from mistreatment or tragedy that overwhelms the human resilience of virtually anyone who suffers them. Combat, rape, being hit by somebody raging, being sexualized early in life, or devastated by some major loss events are not visible from the outside but can easily be relived in the inherent vulnerability of receiving healthcare.

The continuum of hurt can be seen this way, from a nurse's snub or a missed birthday, to a romantic failure, to violent abuse, combat, rape, child neglect, torture, and domestic violence.

GOALS OF SPIRITUAL CARE TO CONSIDER

- Quiet, seemingly timeless personal presence almost always feels supportive.

- Listen to fear and anger for hints of the hurt that lies beneath them.

- Convey empathy regarding specific hurts as stories emerge.

- Gently and only as the patient is ready, bring perspective on the person's own part in the hurtful occurrence.

- Validate tears, accept them, or consider confronting them on occasions when they feel manipulative.

- Evaluate the victimhood.

- Evaluate the discouragement and consider referral for evaluation of depression.

7. NEEDING EMPOWERMENT

As clinicians know, especially those working in emergency care settings, there is a considerable segment of society that has established a dependent personality style and feel chronically victimized. In addition, there is a widespread phenomenon among many other people in which they lose their capacity to cope when thrust into a crisis situation. During periods of regression—unconsciously taking refuge in early life coping behavior such as temporary hysteria, decisional incapacity, teary collapse, or near total helplessness—a person needs the extended presence of a calm and genuinely interested person to gain back his/her ability to meet the foul realities of human living. Inquiry into how the person has coped with similar situations in the past, instruction on the limitations of healthcare and its necessary triage priorities, and exploration of the person's attitudes towards prayer can be tried, as a caregiver hopes for a greater capacity to care for one's own self to re-emerge inside the person in crisis.

GOALS OF SPIRITUAL CARE TO CONSIDER

- Explore the patient's ways of dealing with past similar situations.

- Further orient the patient to the medical realities of his particular situation, or procure that clarifying orientation by another appropriate professional.

- Discover any supportive people that may be available to the patient.

- Instruct the patient on the limitations of healthcare regarding the medical situation.

- Invite prayer to facilitate change in responsibility from outside to inside the patient—i.e. what one can do vs. what one cannot.

Axis 2: Five major loss needs

Axis 2 encompasses the ways in which major loss affects the human personality and, as a life theme, contributes to actually shaping that personality over the entire span of a lifetime. To some degree life is experienced as receiving specific assets without choosing them—a uniquely configured body, a few people along the direct line of reproduction, and some others we come to deeply value, as well as an array of various other entities of personal value such as pets, places, and artifacts. Human experience also includes having to part permanently with all of these, one at a time, and then eventually all together with the last flicker of life itself. How we meet those losses constitutes a history of our grieving that reactivates, quite unpredictably, throughout our lives.

This theme of a person's grieving can easily bob to the surface during hospitalization at a real threat of another such major loss. Hospitalized people often experience bits of grief of previous losses that remain unresolved—striving to be "solved again" by reminiscence, reflection, storytelling, and sometimes rumination and even perseverance. For most of us that process progresses more effectively in conversation with at least one other human being who has skill and motivation to personally listen and facilitate the verbal sharing that finds its own pace, like gestation and friendship.

Five clusters of major losses make up Axis 2: current or recent loss, prior loss, dying, radical change in function or appearance such as from stroke or disfiguring/disabling injury, and estrangement.

8. CURRENT/RECENT LOSS

This issue is one of the primary reasons to use chaplains in medical facilities. Major loss is a primary way in which people starkly realize that there are powers beyond us all, regardless of how this patient conceptualizes what or who that power is.

Needing to begin incorporating into your life history the new realization that somebody or something important to you is suddenly gone, or about to be, constitutes a universal spiritual need. Rendering us clearly powerless to stop the loss, those times make the fact of transcendent power obvious. The personal processes that tend to follow major loss, now collectively called grieving, progress at their own pace. They can partially be facilitated by interpersonal care in the window of the first few hours after the loss. The need of survivors is often for human interaction with a person who is familiar with the process and how to allow its unfolding while quietly encouraging it towards verbal processing, shared reminiscence, immediate planning, and communal remembrance. Grieving styles differ greatly among the individuals involved, and the early grieving process can either consolidate warmth or exacerbate conflict among them.

GOALS OF SPIRITUAL CARE TO CONSIDER

- Quiet presence, with only unpressured words.

- Allow expressions that may initially feel bizarre.

- Pick up on patient or family comments that can initiate a bit of reminiscence.

- Resist informing too easily, before really listening.

- Be silent, but not for too long.

- Gently validate feelings about the loss, and tears if they start.

- Pick up on changes in the communal grieving, towards planning.

- Stay alert for an interest in prayer, sacrament, the presence of a specific trusted spiritual leader, and respond prescriptively.

9. PRIOR LOSS

Healthcare settings tend to raise to consciousness previous major losses, with their accompanying warm, sad, loving, and disappointing memories. Needing to share feelings and reminiscences about a major loss experienced long ago calls for a good listener to recognize and then respond with gentle use of a few focused and compelling questions, giving the impression that endless time is available. Such remedial grieving generally takes no longer than 20 minutes and provides care that is not likely to be forgotten.

Some myths about grieving processes inhibit this care. Belief that grieving can be done thoroughly, once and for all, and then the griever will be OK, is one such assumption. Belief that vigorous emotional expression is essential to a healthy grief process may be another. A griever may emote and process with one person and to others he looks like he has never grieved. Despite the hundreds of books written on the grieving process since C.S. Lewis's *A Grief Observed* in 1961, the care of prior loss in healthcare settings still limps.

GOALS OF SPIRITUAL CARE TO CONSIDER

- Use gentle, focused questions to draw out and validate expressions and reminiscences from people about their major life losses.

- Support and listen.

- Query about how it has felt to speak openly about the prior loss.

- Consider referral for further grieving.

10. DYING

Receiving radical new awareness that a condition is very likely terminal will probably always remain pivotal to a life. Our human need to accomplish final goodbyes and "last things" in preparation for our own death is a classical spiritual care issue that is now being increasingly well addressed by hospice and palliative care professionals. A large percentage of people still die without that specialized care and this need can be appreciably met by at least one savvy helper who has learned to: 1) artfully initiate conversations in which that process can be assisted; 2) listen carefully and personally; 3) patiently bring wisdom and perspective to conversations about dying, patient's religious questions and concerns, what might be ahead after death, and the central events of a person's entire life. The timing of these conversations needs to be in consultation with other IDT members.

The need to say goodbye is often not recognized by patients or family members until it is suggested by a caring outsider. Then there can be a slightly confusing time when one wonders just how to do that. A chief characteristic of hospice programs has been that patients and family members are surrounded by caregivers who are at least a little familiar with that process. Saying goodbye well is essentially communicating clearly what a given person has meant to you, highlighting the best moments of the relationship. It is highly personal, starkly and softly direct, and focused on genuine appreciation for what specifically has generated gratefulness. It is surprisingly brief, boldly focused, and can look easy. It also contributes to the lives of both people involved in ways that will likely never be forgotten. It is a major component of the dying role, a new way of being, that is generated in a person who has developed reasonably well as a person and who becomes clearly aware of his imminent demise.

Assistance with saying goodbye can be accomplished sometimes in one session, helping a person to identify people with whom they want closure and helping to prepare them to do so verbally. So easy to avoid, this project consolidates the place of the two people in one another's lives, and contributes to the peaceful death of one and the grief path of the other.

GOALS OF SPIRITUAL CARE TO CONSIDER

- Notice a person's reminiscences and facilitate those memories into periods of life review.

- Clarify which people the patient selects to receive a goodbye. It generally needs to be a short list.

- Assure the patient that not including everyone is acceptable and even necessary.

- Suggest a time of reflection on just what words to use, only "rehearsing" when requested to do so.

- Offer to facilitate the conversation.

- Offer to debrief the goodbye efforts afterwards. Assist the goodbye needs of family members prescriptively as well.

DYING ALONE?

Introduction

I did my initial rounds in pre-surgery from 6:45–7:20 a.m. I went back to the CPE room and charted. Afterwards, one of the chaplains asked me to just stay and do pre-surgery for the morning. I saw two or three patients and then went into the B-2 room; it was now 8:41 am. The curtain was open and the lights were turned off and the 62-year-old man was lying on his side and looked very uncomfortable. His head was almost off the pillow and bent at such an angle towards his chest that he looked like a contortionist. He was extremely frail and having a difficult time breathing. There was no one around, no family and no friends. The patient looked vulnerable and very anxious. I had looked at his chart and he was going into surgery for a gastrostomy tube insertion. I thought to myself, "Why isn't there someone in the room with this patient?"

Analysis

After visiting the rest of the patients for pre-surgery, I went back to the CPE training room to chart. My visit with R was still on my mind, and while charting I decided to look at R's file to find out what was going on besides the gastrostomy tube surgery. R had cancer, and also had cachexia, which is described as a syndrome of progressive weight loss, anorexia, and persistent erosion of host body cell mass in response to a malignant growth. I felt nauseous; I felt consumed with anxiety over R, and how could such a sweet man have all this going on, and where was his support system? His chart said he had a sister in the area; where was she? I realized I was jumping to conclusions and that I did not have any reason to do that, and what was I going to accomplish anyway? The chart also revealed he had "None" written under "Spiritual requests." I listened to my inner voice from CPE again, and got out his file, and decided there was little else to do; end-of-life care had already been started. Let it go!

The very next night I was on call for the night. Again, one of the chaplains gave me my "marching orders" and off I went. My job was to see the not-yet-seen patients. I almost made it to the first patient when the trauma pager went off, once, no twice, then someone was being taken off of life support, then another trauma. It's going to be a long night (I said to myself); it's only 5:00. Things finally settled down, at least for the moment, and I decided to make rounds to see if any of the patients were still awake. It was 9:50 in the evening and the patient in room 345 was still watching TV. I went in, introduced myself and visited for a few minutes. We had a nice visit. I left and decided to see if anyone else was awake. I glanced into the room next door, room 133. Boy, that guy looked familiar (I thought to myself), but I kept walking. It dawned on me about 30 seconds later, it was R. I decided to go back and see if he was awake and to see how his surgery went. As I entered the room, R looked much like he did from our pre-surgery visit except he was facing the opposite direction, still had the same expression and still had the bent neck. The lights were still off as well.

Chart note

The patient is a 62-year-old, lonely, emaciated male who cannot communicate well and is having a difficult time breathing. He was surgically having a gastrostomy tube inserted, so he could get nourishment and continue with end-of-life care. The patient could only nod his head and whisper to communicate his concerns, and was choking and gasping for air. After having respiratory treatment he calmed down and relaxed. I stayed with the patient and held his hand and read to him until the surgery team came. I hope to follow up with patient, as I have concerns for him being all by himself with no support.

Suggested improvements

The patient is a 62-year-old lonely, emaciated male who is dying alone. He has time breathing as he awaits a surgical procedure to allow him the nourishment needed to continue end-of-life care. He could only nod his head and whisper to communicate his concerns, and he was choking and gasping for air. After respiratory treatment he calmed down and relaxed. I stayed with the patient and held his hand and read to him until the surgery team came.

- *Goal*: I hope to follow up with patient, as I have concerns for him being all by himself with no support. Contact patient's sister to apprise her of his condition and encourage her involvement in his dying process if she is able.

- *Goal*: Provide as much calm human presence as possible as long as patient can benefit.

RATIONALE FOR SUGGESTED IMPROVEMENTS
While this note communicates the chaplain's care quite well, it can be improved by starkly naming the man's dying upfront. He also could take and record more responsibility to help include the man's family in his final care.

11. LIFE ADJUSTMENT

Adjusting to a radical change of appearance or function that is reversible and possibly permanent, challenges the human spirit to retain what resilience and life satisfaction is still available. Accidents, strokes, combat wounds, violent attacks and even events in the mostly gradual physical and mental deterioration from aging and chronic conditions, demand energy and a level of surrender to the limitations of life. Interpersonal care of this need, individually or in groups, can help a person to begin developing a new and necessary style of living.

GOALS OF SPIRITUAL CARE TO CONSIDER

- Hear the stories of the events and progression of the debilitating process as fully as possible.

- Explore the person's religious heritage and current attitudes/practices as possible sources of meaning and purpose for a new future.

- Validate staff insistence on moving forward with rehabilitative efforts in spite of pain, lethargy, and other forms of resistance.

- Consider directly engaging about the future changes that will be likely, encouraging courage and possibly suggesting an ongoing rehabilitative counseling relationship.

- Engage the person frequently if possible to follow the process and tune in to how recent developments are affecting her spirit.

- Stay alert for the person's reflective efforts to find a positive perspective on the decline.

AGING OUTDOORSMAN

Introduction

As I entered B's room, I first saw a man around age 60 sitting up on the hospital bed and looking very alert. It was clear that he had been having a stressful morning—he looked wary and a little bit anxious at first. He had short, graying hair and a matching moustache, and looked very healthy for someone in a hospital bed. There had been some commotion outside this man's room earlier in the day, and I was curious about what had happened to prompt the gathering of docs and nurses I had seen earlier.

Upon entering the room, I was struck by B's attention to me. He had been watching me approach from outside his room, and when I walked in he greeted me immediately. It seemed as though he was trying to maintain some control over his space, even though he couldn't do anything like shut the door. I felt at first like an intruder, but that feeling quickly evaporated after we began talking.

Analysis

B suffers from arterial fibrillation and bleeding ulcers, but does not seem to let this slow him down. He has been hospitalized a couple of times recently, but is a very cheerful and engaging man, even when he has to come in to the hospital. During this conversation B was mostly upbeat and easygoing, especially when he was talking with his friend S, but underneath the calm and collected exterior lie some worries about his general health starting to decline. He is very passionate about the outdoors, and worries that his health will not allow him to continue working and playing out in nature. I got the impression that he is a man of strong principles, and he explicitly expressed admiration for Christian values and morals. I don't think he considers himself to have a personal relationship with God, but nonetheless he can perceive the sacred in his wife's faith and in nature.

As I entered B's room I was making a conscious effort to be cheerful and upbeat because I wasn't sure what had happened that had necessitated the pack of docs and nurses that had been in there before me, and I didn't want to add to his potential worries by looking serious and somber. This quickly turned out to be unnecessary however, as B was in good spirits and immediately engaged me in conversation. As we chatted, I realized that he was keeping our conversation on a surface level, and so I tried to take things to a more emotional level by asking him about faith. I was first taken off guard by the arrival of his friend S, and I felt awkward at first standing in the room while they talked, but I was soon at ease. As it turned out, S's arrival was a great source of information, because not only was B much more willing to talk about health concerns with him, but I had visited S's wife who was the patient in the next room before this visit without realizing it. I learned more about her situation from staying with B and S because she had not been very willing to talk to me earlier. I don't think I did a very good job being reflective; the tone of my comments seems much more supportive and questioning in nature, with the possible exception of one reflective comment.

Chart note

The patient is a man in his mid-60s, who is a hunting guide by profession. He is passionate about the outdoors and is an avid fisherman in his recreational time. He is a very straightforward communicator—he was willing to speak with me openly and honestly when communicating his concerns about his health condition. He spoke of an episode where his vision was impaired for a short time. This was a very scary experience because of his livelihood—the patient asked me, "What the hell good is a blind hunting guide?" I will follow up with him in the days to come to see how he is coping with his current hospitalization.

Suggested improvements

The patient is a man in his mid-60s who is a hunting guide by profession, passionate about the outdoors and an avid fisherman in his recreational time. I visited with him in the presence of his friend who appears to be a significant resource to him. He was able to speak with me openly about an episode in which his vision was impaired for a short time, saying, "What the hell good is a blind hunting guide?" He is likely facing a major life adjustment as he transitions from a highly enjoyable profession to an unknown future due to his heart condition, his declining eyesight, his need for income, and his aging. The patient communicates quite openly and directly when engaged directly.

- *Goal*: I will follow up this conversation to encounter him about his state in life and the adjustment he is facing.

---

12. ESTRANGEMENT

Illness or injury often bring to the fore reconsideration of open interpersonal conflicts that have distanced and even estranged people from one another. This need occurs in hospitals when patients and family members seek to reunite with specific people who have either felt or caused major relationship hurts in the past. What a patient then needs is a process of verbal processing with an interpersonally skilled person, to decide either to attempt reconciling on the one hand, or accept the nasty truth that one has already done all one can to bring reconciliation with the other.

GOALS OF SPIRITUAL CARE TO CONSIDER

- Hear the story of the estrangement and its causing events from the patient's point of view as thoroughly as possible.

- Ask whether, if the estranged one would call the patient at this point, he would accept the call.

- If the answer is yes, ask if the patient would want the caregiver to call the estranged one. If so, facilitate the conversation.

- If the patient refuses to accept the initiative that would come from the estranged one, continue with any other issues.

- If the estranged one refuses to be in contact with the patient, suggest that the patient has done all he can to resolve the relationship.

SAD CANCER ESTRANGEMENT

Introduction

As I was finishing up some charting, a man who was walking the hall came up to me. I introduced myself as a chaplain and he then asked me to come and visit his wife. He told me that she was having a real hard time in the hospital, and needed someone to come see her. The husband was concerned that his wife would start refusing treatment soon.

As I approached the room, I could hear the patient crying from the hallway. I walked in to find a woman in her late 60s lying supine in the hospital bed with tears streaming down her face. She was accompanied by a nurse who looked like she was at her wits end. The husband came back into the room with me and took his place in the chair on the far wall of the room.

Analysis

When I walked in, I immediately sensed that E was looking for comfort of some sort. There was no hostility in her eyes, only pain and sorrow, so I felt comfortable right away kneeling down at her bedside. E's experience of God has been distant at best in recent years. She told me that God hates her, that He is punishing her, and that she was a bad person. I believe that E. feels abandoned by God at various points throughout her life, and that this contributes greatly to the difficulty she is facing in treatment. There is a great deal of strife among her children; she is estranged from two of her three daughters. They haven't spoken in years, and there are grandchildren whom E. has never gotten the chance to meet. By the end of the encounter E. was in a much better mood, even giving me a rather weak and watery smile. She was feeling more optimistic about her upcoming procedures, and even joked a little with her husband. I wonder whether she has any further emotional or mental ailments that might have exacerbated the situation with the nurse that morning.

Before I walked in, I was feeling a bit apprehensive. I could hear E crying from several doors down the hall, and wasn't sure I was ready for this visit. When I walked in, though, I wasn't particularly uncomfortable. I knelt down and remained there for the duration of the visit, and this really seemed to help me to connect with E right from the start. I did fumble a few times during our conversation. There was a stretch of time when no matter what subject I asked about, I accidentally brought up some other tragedy in E's life, almost like I was jumping directly from landmine to landmine. I was aware of a very deep desire in myself throughout the visit for E to say out loud that she didn't want to die, and this desire began in me immediately after I heard her say that she did. That desire, I think, is what drove me to keep asking and keep looking for some safe conversational ground to land on, so that I could have a place from which to start persuading E that her death really wasn't the solution.

Chart note

This is a married woman in her late 60s who was crying and disconsolate when I met her. She is in a great deal of spiritual/emotional pain, due to many different calamities occurring seemingly at once. The patient has been undergoing treatment for cancer for several years, and has experienced a great deal of loss and strife in both her family of origin and among her children. The patient was sad but willing to engage in conversation. I spoke with the patient for about 20 minutes, was able to get her calmed down and cooperative, and plan to follow up later in the afternoon, if time permits. I plan also to coordinate with the night chaplain to continue care for her into the following day, if necessary.

Suggested improvements

This is a married woman in her late 60s whose husband told me he is afraid she will decide to refuse treatment soon. I saw her at his request. She was crying and disconsolate when I first met her, telling me about her years of cancer treatment and a great deal of loss in her family, including the estrangement of two of her three children and some grandchildren she has never met. She calmed some as we talked.

The patient needs help processing the estrangement towards decisions about how to address it and either improve it or reconcile herself to it, possibly through counseling. Her husband could benefit from some brief counseling to help him care for himself while supporting her.

Both could benefit from exploring their religious heritage and current beliefs/practices as possible sources of support, meaning and purpose for this crucial time of their lives.

- *Goal*: I will follow up to help them consider these directions for their future.

Axis 3: Five religious and spiritual practice needs

The highly complex morass of religious history, belief, and practice that now mixes uniquely in virtually every person, from atheist to zealot, can be organized into a few fundamental spiritual needs frequently seen in hospitalized people. Oversimplified as this may seem, it is necessary in order to care briefly and practically for all people when they need guidance and support from their own array of beliefs and practices during challenging times.

A pragmatic summary of the evolution of religion can serve as background here. A few highly reflective individuals have come along at various times in history who became passionate about the human spirit, devised unique ways to support it, and eventually taught those beliefs and practices to followers. Moses, Muhammad, Jesus, and Gautama Buddha were some of the most influential. Their bodies of teaching and practice have evolved into the world's major religions that continue to guide and sustain millions of people.

On the other hand, the human element in religious leadership has sometimes been injurious to the people they proposed to help. The immense vulnerability of people relative to transcendence and the basic unanswered questions of an uncontrollable world have been used to exploit people and have also compelled some to contend with one another regarding what seems like ultimate truth, even to the point of combat.

In clinical practice this highly complex global situation shows itself in any patient's unique array of highly charged values and practices that lies partially visible just beneath their self-presentation. For purposes of rendering the resultant complexity of needs into imperfect but useable form, it can be divided into five specific spiritual needs: religious support, spiritual validation, spiritual counseling, relief from regrets and instructions.

13. RELIGIOUS SUPPORT

The traditional, most basic religious need is for an experience of the transcendent as personal, near, and "on one's side" in solidarity against life's unwanted events. Mere words do not fill this need. It is a felt experience that is called for. Practically speaking, praying is *integrating authentic and relatively intense emotion with words addressed to an image of benign transcendence.* Despite being addressed to a deity that is obviously not always able or willing to get us what we want, the human process of self-expressive prayer shows enough benefit to enough people that it can be encouraged and facilitated as useful in most healthcare situations. Research shows that an overwhelming percentage of patients would even like their physician or nurse to pray with them on occasion.[5]

Classically there are four different kinds of prayer: *asking* for something or help in getting it; *gratefulness*, that natural, almost exuberant response to beauty and good fortune; apologizing and *asking for forgiveness* for the regrets of actions or neglects that continue to haunt us; and *praise*, expressing appreciation for transcendence seen as personal and the unfathomable beauty of the universe overall. Added to these could be a fifth—protest prayer: Job's scolding of God; Tevye's complaints about his perceived undeserved misfortunes; and more contemporarily, the nasty soliloquy of Josiah Bartlett in the shuttered national cathedral on the *West Wing* TV series. All of these can be parts of prayer with patients after listening to their stories and reflecting their apparently deepest concerns in a spontaneous prayer.

Religious support is not limited, however, to the classically central action of prayer. Religious rituals, sacraments, symbols, readings, dietary convictions, repeatedly verbalized beliefs, and ways of wording morals and values, all can be promoted in healthcare settings wherever a given patient is familiar with and open to them. Religious practice has the potential to calm the human spirit, giving an impression that uncontrollable events and consequences are in caring and powerful hands, lending some measure of acceptance of whatever actually occurs.

---

5   There are many studies on prayer in the US literature. A 2014 Pew Research Center study found that 55 percent of respondents said they pray at least once a day, and over a third attend religious services weekly. (Available at www.pewforum. org/2015/11/03/chapter-2-religious-practices-and-experiences/#private-devotions, accessed on September 24, 2016.) Regarding the notion that physicians should pray with patients in various situations, respondents generally disagreed with that as an obligation. Still, some patients actually say they would prefer that physicians inquire about their spiritual and religious lives and offer to pray with them. (See B. Schlawin (2014) *Patient Preference for Physician Prayer in Medical Situations*. Cedar Falls, IA: UNI Scholar Works. Available at http://scholarworks.uni.edu/cgi/viewcontent. cgi?article=1146&context=hpt, accessed on May 18, 2016.)

GOALS OF SPIRITUAL CARE FOR CONSIDERATION

- Since this need is for an experience of a positive transcendence, the primary goal is to provide that experience with the patient as effectively as possible. Shared prayer in various forms is by far the most common such intervention. Sacred rituals, formal confession, conversation with a preferred spiritual leader, and attendance at communal worship events are others.

14. SPIRITUAL VALIDATION

Not all spiritual beliefs and practices are directly related to the world's great religious traditions. Today the Internet is populated by thousands of spiritual leaders who offer (or sell) teachings and practices that are tried and followed by millions who loosely associate with one another to reinforce each other's human spirits. And not all the ways people nourish their human spirits with defined practices and belief fall into what is even broadly called religious.

In a healthcare milieu, supporting what seems to work for a given person's human spirit maintenance often has the best chance of actually being helpful. Spiritual modalities that seem weird to one clinician may be the glue that holds together a patient's personality under terrible circumstances. When a person talks with enthusiasm about whatever seems to delight him, from raising rescue dogs and playing rugby to practicing Wiccan and dancing with a grandchild, the most fitting need is for validation. When a spiritual leader confirms the value of such a spiritual modality it shores up a method of dealing with the uncontrollable that works and is probably needed for the current crisis.

On the other hand, when a spiritual modality appears to be destructive to persons or is impeding professional care, intricate negotiating may be necessary. Sometimes the result will be for the clinician to accept the limitations of assuaging religious beliefs and surrendering to what seems like ridiculous waste. At other times, however, the common good of the healthcare community may need to be protected. In such complex and difficult situations, well-developed healthcare ethics committees make determinations about what is best in a given situation when no good solution is possible. A spiritual caregiver then considers making a referral to that committee. When even that committee fails to be up to effectively engaging the situation, a spiritual caregiver remains with the patient's heart and family as long as possible.

GOALS OF SPIRITUAL CARE FOR CONSIDERATION

- Discern whether the method of spiritual nurturance described by the patient actually benefits him or hinders his spirit in this situation.

- Validate it as fitting for that person, or intricately intervene to question its potential harm to him.

- Provide a calm human presence as long as possible or as long as it is accepted.

15. SPIRITUAL COUNSELING

Religious and spiritual leadership have not always been helpful to people's human spirits. Sometimes the best religious teaching a patient has received, whether in childhood, youth, or adulthood, has never been incorporated into that person's life. At other times religious leadership has failed to provide adequate direction and guidance at pivotal life events. Many people have even found in religious teaching a mixture of insight on the one hand and exploitation on the other. What presents itself in a clinical setting then consists of a history of insufficient teaching rather than useful practices, rebuke rather than support, and propaganda rather than insightful teaching.

Wounding of the human spirit has often resulted from engaging both organized and independent spiritual leaders. Many patients bring to the hospital or clinic a confusing history and patchy array of convictions about what might really work for them spiritually.

Spiritual wounding hides, however. Like most of spirituality (and iatrogenic occurrences in medicine) it is not directly observable most of the time. In healthcare, religious wounded-ness is most likely to surface in the presence of spiritual leaders whose manner reminds them on some level of the worst events of their religious history. They may ask a question brought on by their hospitalization that indicates a deeper confusion beneath the surface, such as, "Is suicide a quick ticket to hell?" or "If I stop dialysis is that suicide?" A patient's sharply critical religious comment in the context of a mostly social conversation also may be revealing this painful or enraging disenchantment with religion. Hospitalization can bring the chance meeting with a caregiver or spiritual leader who seems to care about him as a human being, not merely as another potential sheep in the flock.

This need is found anywhere on a continuum between curious questions on the one hand and hostile, reactive iconoclasm resulting from serious past religious abuse on the other.

GOALS OF SPIRITUAL CARE FOR CONSIDERATION

Regarding religious wounding:

- Hear the stories of the offensive events as thoroughly as possible.

- Help the person distinguish between one harmful individual or system on the one hand, and a positive transcendence on the other.

- Mostly refrain from defending or promoting any particular religious system.

- Consider referral to a pastoral counselor or other widely trusted religious leader.

Regarding religious questions:

- Hear the concern and elicit the reasons it is being asked at this particular time.

- Provide a context for the religious principles involved, as accurately as possible.

- Consider referral to another appropriate religious or spiritual leader.

16. RELIEF FROM REGRETS

Sometimes referred to as "the mother of all spiritual issues," guilt lies beneath the conscious surface of many patients who quietly feel punished by their condition for previous behavior or neglect of fundamental responsibilities. They are compelled to believe they may deserve what they are suffering, rather than becoming resentfully convinced that they don't. Personal isolation can result from the fact that large strains of our society brush aside guilt as an unfortunate "trip" that only immature people take.

In truth, however, like physical pain that signals bodily injury or dysfunction, natural guilt is a self-criticizing inner sense that we've caused hurt to somebody else, to a particular group or to society in general. It is innate in humanity, except for in those who have been treated very badly as children, what some call sociopaths or psychopaths. A realistic level of guilt is humanly healthy but may need assuaging when it burgeons during hospitalization.

Shame, on the other hand, is generally distinguished from guilt though they sometimes coexist. Guilt is about our behavior, and shame is about being somehow inadequate as a person. Clinically shame lowers the eyes so as not to meet another's gaze. Shame is likely related to the fact that we all grow up little when most people around us are big and easily complete simple tasks that are still mysterious to us. Too much shaming in the family of origin context sets some children up for a life totally oriented around blaming—either oneself or somebody else.

The classical Roman Catholic sacrament of confession was intended to relieve guilt relatively easily, and it is still used that way by some people. Restorative rituals in some African tribes similarly address serious behavioral transgressions to absolve the immense guilt that collects in a delinquent person's core. The original founders of Alcoholics Anonymous discovered the same need in people whose addiction had propelled them onto a cycle of guilt from impulsive, selfish lives. Those early recovering alcoholics needed a way for themselves and others to deal with the massive guilt of years of drinking behavior. They worded the Fifth Step[6] to promote the process of unburdening oneself through catharsis or sharing, relating in verbal detail all that they had done that they now regret.

In the clinical setting some professionals have become accustomed to unpredictable events of listening to people's blurted renditions of regretted incidents, actions, attitudes, and neglect, brought on by the self-reflective vulnerability of needing healthcare. If they listen and tease out whatever detail of regretted incidents the patient needs to share, they function briefly as confessors.

Confessing, simply admitting guilt in appropriately detailed form, is only the beginning of the classical forgiveness ritual however. Another key piece of it includes a human being listening and declaring forgiveness by the Deity and the human community, classically called absolution. The most common mistake made by student chaplains and some veterans as well is moving too quickly to absolution, truncating the spiritually therapeutic value of the confessing itself. Making nice assertions that "God forgives you" spouted too quickly short-circuits the pain of sharing what really hurts inside the guilty person. A measure of that pain is necessary.

GOALS OF SPIRITUAL CARE FOR CONSIDERATION

- Elicit concrete detail of regretted behavior.

- Maintain strict confidentiality, even generalizing in chart notes to mercifully cover the exact nature of the behavior and its worst details.

---

6   Step Five states, "[We] Admitted to God, to ourselves, and to another human being the exact nature of our wrongs" (Alcoholics Anonymous 1953, pp.55–62).

- Linger enough to allow related, or even unrelated, regrets to rise to the surface of consciousness as well.

- Refrain from either moralizing or too easy normalizing of the regretted behavior. Neither works.

- Validate forgiveness by the Deity or at least yourself within the limits of your own beliefs.

17. INSTRUCTION

The orienting information and medical education received by patients from healthcare professionals is indeed a kind of spiritual care. Increasing a person's medical literacy by instruction from nurses and physicians tends to calm the human spirit when accurately and humanly conveyed. A similar need is for education, or better understanding of what one may have heard somewhere about spirituality and various other care modalities but which never became effectively useable in a given person's life. In clinical settings human spirits can be prescriptively bolstered by clarifying or augmenting instruction on spiritual teachings and other complementary modalities designed to affect the spirit positively. Some of the most common needs for instruction include:

- *medical ethics*: the need for explanation of sets of principles that give direction when complexities keep any single effective direction from emerging as obviously best

- *advanced directives*: documents that clarify to the extent possible what treatments a given person may want to exclude when she becomes unable to speak for herself

- *chemical dependence*: at a specific point in encountering a possible substance abuse problem, a person suspected of problem usage of mood altering chemicals can benefit from learning about addiction and how some such other people begin to find recovery

- *rituals and sacraments*: combining words with reverent actions has been helpful to the human spirit for thousands of years

- *meditation*: the opposite of rumination, meditation holds positive ideas in the mind and MRI researchers seem to be proving that it helps people who practice it well (Newberg and Waldman 2009)

- *devotions*: repetition of earnest sentiment based on spiritual beliefs calms the spirit for some people

- *guided imagery*: facilitated calming and inspiring imaginings have been shown to be beneficial in cancer patients

- *healing touch and other potentially enriching modalities.*

GOALS OF SPIRITUAL CARE FOR CONSIDERATION

Completion of any of the above areas of instruction, and others in which the caregiver is competent, may serve as goals of care for this spiritual need.

Axis 4: Five referral needs

The personal vulnerability inherent in hospitalization can catalyze openness of a patient to receiving assistance for specific, complex and difficult, painful conditions and situations, either pre-existing or emanating from the hospitalization itself, that need specialized help. Any caregiver with skill and experience at referral can assist a patient or family to recognize the serious need and take action to address it. Referral is in itself an art. It requires sensitivity, patience, strategizing, knowledge, preparation, and careful conversation. Interpersonal courage, peer consultation, and practice can improve skills for referring.

Probably the most difficult aspect of the art of referral is to elicit emotion before suggesting the patient seek another form of care. It is actually feeling the pain of the self-sabotaging difficulty that may motivate a person to follow through and actually seek specialized help. Simply suggesting such life-changing help can often be merely copping out on the caregiver role. It is too easy. It doesn't work, even if the patient agrees to the referral. Only rarely will a patient take that help-getting step unless one actually sees the pain on their face while talking about it.

Some common spiritual needs that suggest referral to other forms of care, besides those already mentioned above, include medical ethics confusion, mental illness/addiction, family conflict, advocacy, and love life pain.

18. MEDICAL ETHICS CONFUSION

A profound unsettling of the human spirit occurs when options for treatment become hypercomplex or are seen seriously diminishing in effectiveness. When no healthcare regimen obviously promises to be restorative of the previous level of health and life quality, consultation about the best next step is indicated. Any interdisciplinary team member, including chaplains, may be the first to hear a patient's distress over medical ethics issues. Referral to the unit IDT, a palliative care program, or a functional medical ethics committee can relieve a great deal of this painful confusion.

The rapidly growing specialty of palliative medicine has seen that persistent physical pain is almost always accompanied by the inner suffering of decisional churning, interpersonal conflicts, profound fears, and religious binds. All of those constitute suffering of the human spirit and some lend themselves especially to care by skilled spiritual caregivers. Palliative care teams have been instrumental in developing a team approach to addressing this need, especially in complex cases that include a need for medical palliation. A spiritual caregiver role in palliative care, distinct from the functioning of other clinicians, is evolving along with the specialty.

GOALS OF SPIRITUAL CARE FOR CONSIDERATION

- When any caregiver hears a patient or family member mention feeling a dilemma regarding the efficacy of current treatment, listen as clearly as possible, and stretch to understand the patient's situation.

- Clarify any ethical principles involved to a degree that is within the limitations of your healthcare discipline.

- Assess the need for an appropriate clinician to offer further instruction about the condition and the prognosis.

- Consider calling for a family or ethics committee consultation.

19. MENTAL ILLNESS AND ADDICTION CONCERNS

Helping people understand and manage their mental illnesses remains a major component of the jobs of healthcare clinicians of all disciplines. Caregivers carry a considerable responsibility to participate actively in the vast and complex global project of assisting the 46 percent of the US population that will experience a mental disorder that is at least temporarily disabling in their lifetime. Only an estimated third of the people experiencing the various mood disorders, personality disorders, and other life troubling conditions are getting needed treatment. Clinical settings offer a window of opportunity for referral, and clinicians, including spiritual ones, can continually learn both about the various signs of this need and the intricate processes of referring and treating it.

Addiction challenges the human spirit perhaps as much as any other condition. Treatment programs and Alcoholics Anonymous have shown that for most people recovery includes a major spiritual transformation component. An estimated 11 to 30 percent of people experience problems in major areas of their lives from their own mood-altering chemical usage. A caregiver able to carry on a calm conversation about a patient's own concerns about her/his usage can, although infrequently, make use of the narrow window of hospitalization vulnerability to refer for assessment by a counselor.

In a wide definition of spiritual need, mental illness and addiction must be included. Simply put, the human spirit is what gets depressed in depression and distorted in major anxiety disorders. The fields of psychiatry, psychology, social work, and counseling that have developed in the past 150 years provide help for spiritually painful conditions that were previously impossible to treat. Despite the fact that funding for effective care of mental illness and addictions remains horribly inadequate, the interdisciplinary approach to treatment of addictions remains highly effective when practiced well with a mixture of both previously addicted and never addicted staff members, and close collaboration with movements like Alcoholics Anonymous and its clones aimed at promoting recovery from other addictions.

GOALS OF SPIRITUAL CARE FOR CONSIDERATION
For suspected alcoholism or chemical abuse of patient or family member:

- the primary goal is to see the patient accept assessment by a qualified addiction counselor

- develop a calm conversation about the patient's own concerns about her mood-altering chemical usage (this skill is very difficult to learn)

- maintain that calm conversation as long as it can be tolerated by the patient (and you, the caregiver)

- elicit concrete details about the regretted consequences of usage

- elicit emotions about the consequences of the chemical usage as seen by the patient

- query about previous treatment and the patient's experience of and attitude towards it

- suggest assessment by a qualified and experienced alcoholism or addiction counselor.

For potential mental illness of a patient or family member:

- hear the concerns about the disturbing behavior, affect, inclinations, confusion, or anxiety

- elicit openness of disclosure and convey empathy for the feelings about it

- describe what you understand about the experiences of specific mental illness, within the limits of your own understanding

- consult with IDT staff about your concerns and those of the patient

- suggest assessment by a mental health professional, and arrange for it.

20. LOVE-LIFE PAIN

The need for understanding, advice, or referral about hurt in one's love life is very common among both patients and staff members of hospitals. A person's primary relationship affects and is affected by everything else of significance that happens to him/her. Our human spirit soars when we are in love and tanks when that relationship hurts as much as anything else can hurt. As a major aspect of the spirituality of most people, pain in intimate relationships can often benefit from sharing and encounter about further counseling care.

During a healthcare crisis, the one person most people want to be with them is their current lover-spouse-partner. There are exceptions of course. Presence of one's lover becomes particularly difficult when that person and the patient are currently not on good terms. On the other hand, crisis times can turn out to be opportunities for beginning the difficult process of getting help for the relationship itself if caregivers notice, listen, and respond.

GOALS OF SPIRITUAL CARE FOR CONSIDERATION

- To hear as thoroughly as possible the concerns about the person's love life—recent events, persistent conflict, the health of one's partner, and other struggles of the relationship itself.

- To elicit the emotions about the relationship and its current state.

- To query about how it feels to talk about the current struggles.

- To address the prospects of seeking counseling help for the relationship.

21. ADVOCACY

Regardless of the quality of care they receive, some patients and families begin to feel neglected by the healthcare system or specific caregivers. Sorting out which patients actually need a different kind of care than they are getting from the dependent-style personalities who, sometimes unconsciously, have an insatiable yearning for attention, is an art only experienced caregivers develop.

On the other hand, the healthcare culture easily gets preoccupied with procedures and protocols that then inhibit seeing issues that lie beneath. Some patient issues simply do not fit nicely into caregivers' diagnostic worlds. And iatrogenic issues are real, fairly frequent, and often serious in healthcare facilities.

The word "advocate"—from the Latin "to speak for"—is a concept of what fills a need for those who cannot be expected to realize how or when to speak for themselves. It takes courage for a practitioner of any discipline to speak for a patient to another caregiver in assisting that person to get either basic assistance when being neglected or a different form of care altogether. It also requires astute observation and intricate interaction to help a dissatisfied patient or family better comprehend the limitations of healthcare and its systems.

GOALS OF SPIRITUAL CARE FOR CONSIDERATION

- To hear the feelings about neglect of not receiving the care or form of care needed.

- To hear the dissatisfaction a patient may have with a current caregiver or caregivers.

- To consider instructive input on the limitations of the current treatment situation or of healthcare itself.

149

- To assess the level of "stuck-ness" in a habitual victim role, not assuming that it cannot exist alongside genuine need.

- To volunteer to accompany the patient in her efforts to obtain improvements.

- To prepare the way for an advocacy conversation by informing the target caregiver of the complaint beforehand.

- To follow up after an advocacy conversation for how it was successful for the patient.

22. FAMILY CONFLICT

A patient seeing interpersonal conflict among her family intensifies the vulnerability of hospitalization and can add disgust to whatever else she is feeling. The seriousness of healthcare situations can either cause new family conflict or rekindle previous complex and difficult family issues. The dramatic nature of serious health issues can sometimes heighten the conflict and fuse it into the family culture for decades. But at other times it can act as a catalyst for reconciliation and growing beyond the conflict.

An astute caregiver, as a neutral person who notices the undercurrents of family disagreement and even helps absorb the anger as it arises, may be able to either facilitate the conflict towards eventual resolution, or deftly refer to other caregivers who can. The alarm of hospitalization and major loss lays open vulnerability that becomes an opportunity to change painful relationships that have lain wounded for years.

GOALS OF SPIRITUAL CARE FOR CONSIDERATION

- To confirm the caregiver's impressions of family conflict serious enough to affect patient care and progress.

- To identify the primary family members involved in the conflict.

- To ascertain what are the primary interpersonal dynamics of the conflict.

- To consider querying the patient about the effects of the conflict on her spirit and her healing process.

- To raise the possibility of consultation with an appropriate counselor.

Once a caregiver has recognized the spiritual needs of a patient she faces the next task of representing them to other caregivers face to face and in the patient's chart. Medical record systems, even electronic ones, generally allow for narrative in spiritual care chart notes in one way or another. Defining a specific format for such narrative entries can make it much easier for IDT members to locate, identify, and quickly scan them for salient impressions. Such a format is the subject of the next chapter.

4

Format

A Shape for an Elegant Chart Note

*The best chaplains speak little but listen intently, becoming a
container for all that the patient needs to share and then with great
care sifts through and captures the "pearls" that the larger medical
team need to know and weaves a narrative note that is full of deep
listening, reverence and truth.*

RITA CHARON, MD[1]

A veteran chaplain supervisor has a son who had just finished
medical school. When the budding doctor first got access to patients'
medical records, he would take special notice of those entries written
by chaplains, his father's long-time profession. After a few days he
remarked to his father, "Dad. This one chaplain guy writes the same

---

1   Rita Charon spoke these words to a group of palliative care physicians/practitioners
    including Anne Butler, APRN, during a breakout session of her program on narrative
    medicine at Columbia University Medical Center in September 2006. She was working
    on her book Narrative Medicine: Honoring the Stories of Illness (2008).

thing every time! What's the sense in that?" The fledgling physician and the note-writing chaplain apparently have very different notions of the function of spiritual care chart notes.

If you believe your chart notes are primarily to comply with a policy, to generate numbers for the accountants, contribute to research, support your department's survival, keep your job, or please your director, then checked boxes and filled-in lines will suffice and may even get you accolades. If you believe your notes are written chiefly to your colleague chaplains for follow-up calls, then religious language may be appropriate. But if you know that recording your best spiritual care efforts is also in service to the healing of people and your collaboration with the clinicians who are treating them, then you will scramble to write every note to be descriptive of what you know about that patient's unique inner life, her current personal concerns and her attitudes about her health situation.

As architects have long taught, "form follows function" (Sullivan 1896). A bathroom differs from a kitchen and a bedroom, because they are all designed for different purposes. Similarly, the shape your chart note takes will follow what you think that note is intended to do. As an IDT member you will want a note format that fits the professional culture and essential work of the particular care setting in which you work. Oncology patients will differ from those being treated in neurological rehab, dialysis, and mental health services. Your first note upon meeting a patient or family member will differ from one you write about the same patient three weeks later and on a troubled new admission to a gerontology unit. But all of them will focus some direct comments on the current state of the patient's human spirit, largely gleaned from the stories the patient tells.

A general format for most chaplain notes helps IDT members reading it to anticipate where the salient information will be found and to grasp it quickly. One way to organize a note is to adapt the format used by physicians. Their notes still typically include a line or two followed by several bullet point orders. Doctors are accustomed to seeing that format, as are nurses who need to shape their care to some degree on doctors' orders. The common repetition found in physician notes will be obnoxious in spiritual care notes, however, which are designed to be brief and pointed, and interesting in their reflection of a patient's unique human predicament.

Nurses maintain their own charting style that is illustrated in how they communicate orally in the nursing report that occurs between all shifts. Those brief meetings generally allow little time for discussion. Nurses communicate at shift change, conveying specific information needed to be passed from one shift to another with little rationale given and little explanation of anything. Communication there is crisp, swift, and concrete. When spiritual caregivers are not present at nursing report or physician rounds, they need to communicate about their care in the medical record. To enter effectively into that flow of written data-filled communication, they will need to, as accurately as possible and in commonly understood terms, describe patients and their spiritual needs humanly.

"Capturing the soul" in narrative

In a chart note, a consulting spiritual caregiver is ideally attempting to "capture the soul in writing" of every patient who can still communicate. That means, make your best effort to *summarize succinctly what you know about the immediate life situation of the individual as she sees it, along with conveying your impressions of the current state of that person's human spirit.*

Edward Husserl was a German Jew best known for his philosophical thinking about phenomena—the appearances of things to any given person as distinct from the *noumenon*, how those things actually are. His philosophy, called phenomenology, emphasized the value of accurately describing what one perceives. When we go to "be seen" by a physician, we're asking her to assess the phenomena of our body and put together a reasonable diagnosis and treatments that fit it. She cannot see the total of what is happening in the physical body but operates from lab data, technology images, and direct external observation to make an appraisal based on established criteria and frameworks of understanding various aspects of our physical makeup.

Spiritual caregivers are doing something parallel. We assess the personal, interpersonal, communal, and transcendent relationship phenomena disclosed by a patient and assemble a picture of the state of that person's human spirit. Neither of those assessments, medical nor spiritual, is absolutely comprehensive or exhaustive of the state of either body or soul. But both appraisals are often invaluable to bring understanding enough to guide actions that have a great likelihood of helping that person in the present predicament. Neither always works, and the outcomes of both disciplines mostly fail, as death approaches and nobody can see the afterlife to assess outcomes in any final way.

A spiritual caregiver writing an elegant, and never completely accurate, chart note can be seen engaging in phenomenology, shaping written comments that boldly describe a patient as accurately as possible with relevance to IDT culture in mind. Such a phenomenological description strives to highlight in writing a person's uniqueness in terms that could be recognized by that patient and any other interested careful observer who may read it.

In the phrase "capture the soul," the term "soul" is meant to distinguish serious depth of interaction from social conversation and polite encouragement. Soul implies the sense of "coming from the core" of a person, as in "soul music" or the relationship of "soulmates."[2] The essence of one person discloses itself to another person in the rapport that characterizes spiritual care. The part of a patient conversation that feels more substantive, authentic, and significant can be seen as "soul flow," *an interaction between at least two people relating in a quality*

---

2   Two words evolved from Hebrew (and likely Greek as well) observers of air flowing through the throat. One word, *ruah*, referred to how breathing is an indicator of current emotion or disposition; the other, *nefes*, referred to how without breathing there is no life. *Nefes* could mean the core essence of a person, and then even could mean person. *Ruah* was never used to mean person. These two words are now translated as what we know as spirit (*ruah*) and soul (*nefes*). A spiritual caregiver can thus be seen as watching indicators of feelings, attitudes, or current disposition that then can lead to what is happening in a person's core, or soul (McKenzie 1965, pp.836–839 and 840–845).

collaboration of depth. Grasping what is most salient about such a soulful interaction and conveying it to team members remains an always elusive goal of spiritual care efforts.

The term "narrative" refers to stories, which have been inserting themselves into the practice of several helping disciplines. At least one Ivy League university[3] has established an academic curriculum in narrative medicine to assist medical practitioners to develop the art of turning patient information into stories and using their own life stories as a backdrop to continually improve that art. Indeed there is a small but vibrant movement to better use narrative in the practice of psychology (Kleinman 1989), nursing (Harlan 2014) and social work (Paquin 2009), as well as in pastoral counseling (Sullander 2015) and medicine (Charon 2001; Greenhalgh and Hurwitz 1999; MacGregor 2013). In spiritual care the narrative is intended to highlight the essential humanness of a patient and the unique situation in which that person finds herself. In chart notes those stories need to be lean and succinct reports of the content and meaning of the stories without actually telling them.

Relevant stories of almost any kind better convey the uniqueness of a person than concepts alone. Narratives bring a sense of humanness to people that is not as easily visible in conceptual language. While concepts can be crucial in communicating well-known phenomena such as grieving, estrangement, and life review, they can also become easy words with which to categorize people and thus miss the human-to-human relationship that carries most personal healing potential. There is little pertinent truth in generalizations about people.

A patient narrative is an account of something that happened, is happening, or concerning something for which a person is appreciating, yearning, regretting, or dreading to happen. For chart notes a narrative needs to convey only the patient stories that are brief, clear, and relevant to the current condition of the patient. They imply action, describe movement, and illustrate processes. They bring life to a paragraph. "He gets me" is a colloquial response to a paragraph that has captured at least a portion of a person's soul.

---

3   Columbia University College of Medicine, Narrative Medicine program.

The notion of "capturing the soul" is, however, clearly a metaphor. Spiritual caregivers need to abandon the myth that spiritual assessment actually appraises a person's soul or spirit in any permanent or enduring or even radically accurate way. Any comment about the human spirit of another person remains a speck on the mountain of complexity that makes up any person. We humans never really "get" one another in any comprehensive way. Capturing the soul means only that we make a comment on some significant happening, attitude, stance, or mood that might be relevant to this person in this health situation on this day.

A basic chart note format

A first transformative principle for many newly charting spiritual caregivers is "use sentences." Phrases alone have more difficulty conveying stories and humanness in descriptions of a patient's spirit. Phrases alone may be more efficient but information can be conveyed at least as accurately in thoughtful sentences. The medium of narrative speaks too. It says something like, "This is a real person, unique, admirable, and respectable, so pay attention to her inherent quality and don't abbreviate everything as if she were only a subject of science."

For first-visit patient conversations a chart note format designed to inform busy, decisive, pragmatic, and humanistic physicians and nurses, at this point in history, will include: 1) a *first sentence* often beginning with the patient's basic information and then highlighting what is most striking about this patient at this time; 2) a short paragraph made up of *a few descriptive sentences* that seek to capture the person's unique current personal life situation; and 3) two to four *summary points* of new or immediately relevant information about that patient's experience of and attitudes about her condition, treatment, and the spiritual care that transpired. It should be kept in mind that this format serves as a set of guidelines, not a Procrustean bed of rigidly confining categories.

PRICKLY PEAR: SHARP ON THE OUTSIDE, SWEET ON THE INSIDE

Introduction

I came upon the patient S one day as I was going room to room in the Emergency Department. When I opened up the curtain that was across the entrance I was somewhat taken aback by the sight of this 90-year-old Caucasian woman with rather scraggly, thin, brown/gray hair pulled back on her head, dark sparkling eyes, and a hospital gown that was coming off one shoulder. She looked unkempt and sweaty, like she had not had a shower for some time. My impression was that she was not well cared for. She had been brought to the ED for debility. There were no family members with her at the time I saw her.

Analysis

My visit with patient S was not what one might call "smooth." For me it was a little like rafting a river and discovering, once I got on it, at the start assuming that it's going to be an ordinary, uncomplicated ride, that I would come across hydraulics that would suddenly grab me, suck me into them and then spit me out, shocked. I was struck by an impression that her quick tongue can skewer people as she did me. She also showed surprising depth, astuteness, and deep faith....and a sweetness inside. Part of the patient's sharpness and exasperation can be accounted for by her difficulty hearing, it's true. But some of it is just her, I think. She is staunchly Missouri Synod Lutheran and proud of it. Whatever Martin Luther believed, in her eyes, is the gospel. So she seemed during our visit to stand in opposition to those things she believes Martin Luther did not like, i.e. the Catholic Church and women in church leadership, like me. Yet underneath her appearances and her prickliness is a woman who has suffered a significant amount of loss. Her daughter, who was closest to her and who called her every day, died last month. And her husband of 61 years died three years ago. I experienced her as forgetful and at times, astute, sharp-minded and willing to break out into a Martin Luther hymn at the drop of a hat! I came away from my visit frustrated that I could not spend more time with her, but amazed at who she is.

Chart note

I met the patient while she was still in the ED. She was eating eggs and toast and had eaten most of the other food on the tray. But she complained, "Why do they give me all of this food? I can't eat all this food. So much food goes to waste." When I introduced myself, she seemed agitated, saying, "I am Missouri Lutheran. We don't have female pastors or chaplains." I explained that chaplains serve all different denominations and faiths. She then began to talk, telling me about living in Athens and Italy while her husband served in the Navy. She stated that she is now a navy widow since her husband died. The patient spoke pleasantly as long as she could hear, but became agitated when I spoke to her and she could not hear me. "Open your lips when you talk to me," she demanded at one point. The patient also told me about her 65-year old daughter, who died not long ago. She cried as she recalled how she visited with her each day; she misses her a lot. The patient has other children in the area that she says will be coming to see her when she gets up to the floor. Our visit ended when nursing staff needed to work with her. I will ask another chaplain to follow up with her since she would likely benefit from more processing of her grief.

Suggested improvements

This is a 90-year-old widow who is outspoken, colorful, impulsive, and eccentric, appearing in the ED looking unkempt and frisky. She talks spontaneously, is easily critical of caregivers, (she told me to "open your lips when you're talking to me!") and was reminiscing about living in Europe with her navy husband of 61 years who died several years ago. She cried when talking about her devoted 65-year-old daughter who died two weeks ago. She has other children who she expects to visit her after she is admitted.

- *Goal*: The patient proudly claims solid attachment to the Missouri Synod Lutheran Church and is dedicated to Martin Luther. I will contact a local Lutheran pastor to consider visiting the patient while admitted.

- *Goal*: It is likely that the patient could benefit from further processing her major losses, and I will notify the other chaplain staff to help coordinate further grief work.

RATIONALE FOR SUGGESTED IMPROVEMENTS

- Chatty disclosures don't fit well into the medical record.

- Organizing the information makes reading it more efficient.

- There could be a dispute about the reduced detail of the patient's stories, but brevity is crucial for IDT members.

The all-important first sentence

Excellent first sentences of almost any writing tend to grab the attention of readers and lead them to read on. Great novels have often featured memorable first sentences. Many readers will know, for example, the title and author associated with "Call me Ismael" and "Happy families are all alike; every unhappy family is unhappy in its own way." Perhaps even better known is, "It was the best of times, it was the worst of times..." Sports stories feature the same characteristic. If one doesn't vibrate to the first sentence, after being compelled by the headline, one isn't likely to read the rest of the article.

The classic first sentence of a medical "history and physical" or psychologist's assessment begins with age, gender, marital status, and sometimes work, ethnicity, geography, and reason for admission. It conveys in that opening sentence basic information as a focusing device to get colleagues "into the ballpark" about a particular individual. It concretizes this person as unique. A similar sentence works for spiritual caregivers and is almost indispensable for representing the patient specifically in her current life situation in a first chart note written about her. Such a sentence can touch on several of the primary spiritual arenas of human existence described in Chapter 2.

The best first sentences begin with basic information and end with a brief mini-story that highlights something new, current, or uniquely characteristic about the humanness of the patient. There are several such stories to choose from in virtually every patient with whom depth of rapport is established. A caregiver generally needs to decide which story fits best and most colorfully into the first sentence and consider where to place the other stories that may be relevant. These are some common stories to consider for ending the first sentence.

THE ADMISSION STORY

These stories tell about events that led up to hospitalization and sometimes how the admission took place. While not necessarily essential to medical and nursing care, they can bring out the humanness of a patient. One can consider whether or not most of the staff already know this information before including it in the first sentence.

- Alda is a 69-year-old African American grandmother, *who was accompanied for admission by her nephew after falling and lying, mostly patiently, on her bathroom floor for three hours before he found her.*

- May is a 46-year-old mother and nursing manager, *who suffered her second heart attack while speaking briefly but publically at a department head meeting and was subsequently brought to the ER by her colleagues.*

THE REASON FOR HOSPITALIZATION

What is the story of the medical concern that disturbed the patient's soul seriously enough to motivate her seeking hospital care? This story may be as brief as describing an accident and as complex as summarizing in a phrase a ten-year cancer saga.

- Zelda is an 88-year-old widowed, homebound early Alzheimer's patient, *who was brought in by her cousin who noticed her limping seriously after a minor fall in her kitchen.*

- Zack is a 68-year-old widower and recently retired fixit man, *who became alarmed at blood in his urine for no reason he could think of.*

THE COURSE OF THE ILLNESS/INJURY

This one- or two-sentence narrative may include the long-term development of a medical issue or a series of past events, and recent incidents that are vivid and concerning enough to put together in a shared story.

- Maxine is a 52-year-old grade school teacher, *who tells of her constant fatigue from two years of various treatments for her worsening cervical and uterine cancer.*

- Jacob is a 67-year-old married combat veteran and father, *who recounts many medical events over the past 15 years, including his resentment over some treatments at another facility that have gone awry.*

THE PATIENT'S CURRENT MOOD OR ATTITUDE

Clinicians can be quite interested in the patient's thoughts, feelings, and attitudes, especially towards their medical condition and their caregivers, both the professional and the personal ones (i.e. family and friends). Ways that the "patient experience" is assessed makes these particularly relevant to practitioners tuned into their own and their unit's patient satisfaction scores.

- Susan is a 58-year-old grandmother, *who was musing about a time now boldly approaching when she may need to terminate dialysis.*

- Abe is a 36-year-old married mechanic, *who says he regularly considers "doing anything I can" to stop what he experiences as intractable pain.*

SOMETHING HAPPENS WHEN WE GATHER

Introduction

Summoned to see the patient, by patient request at 7:00 p.m., but had two urgent pages (MVA and parents in PICU requesting prayers for their dying baby), so it was just 9:00 p.m. when I was able to respond to the patient request for a visit. I decided to see if the patient was still awake. As I approached the room, I could hear the patient speaking with her nurse. I knocked and introduced myself, acknowledged the hour and asked if it was too late for a visit. The room was dimly lit, and I observed the patient, a 53-year-old woman of African–Caribbean descent sitting up in bed. She smiled and invited me in. She appeared fatigued and stated that she had been in pain. We spent about 20 minutes together talking primarily about the important people in the patient's life and her relationship with God.

Analysis

The patient was tired, sick, nauseous, and alone, seeking comfort and connection. She warmly welcomed the visit and was able to share some important moments in her life story—the deaths of her parents, the birth of her son, and some of her spiritual history and longings.

The chaplain accepted the patient's invitation to come close, both literally and spiritually, to enter into the experience of sitting quietly in the dark, waiting for what stories needed to be shared. Although at the end of the encounter many pieces of information were still unknown (diagnosis, prognosis, expected length of stay), the chaplain felt grateful for the chance to sit with the patient in her uncertainty (patient's and chaplain's) and to find God in the space between chaplain and patient.

Chart note

Patient admitted with nausea and vomiting, requested chaplain visit. The patient has a long history of caring for other family members and now finds herself ill and in need of care. The patient grew up in Trinidad where she made connection to both Roman Catholic and Baptist churches, searching for church community in this city area. Offered prayer and pastoral support. The patient would like a visit from chaplain tomorrow, referral made.

Suggested improvements

This is a 53-year-old single woman of African–Caribbean descent who communicated warmly and openly, appearing to be tired, sick, nauseous, and alone. She shared easily about the major losses in her life and her current situation of an isolated existence, having been in this area for 20 years but having no significant connections here now. Her long history of caring for other family members leaves her now with nobody to accompany her in her own hospitalization and current life. The patient thinks a lot as she continues to grieve about her deceased son, who was a major source of support for her. The chaplain sat in the dark with the patient as she shared extensively about herself and her life.

- *Goal*: The patient requested another chaplain visit tomorrow when she hopes to have more energy, which I arranged.

RATIONALE FOR SUGGESTED IMPROVEMENTS

- More detail enriches the representation of the patient–chaplain relationship.

- Clarity about the closeness of the chaplain–patient relationship, the human-to-human care the patient is receiving, is reassuring to some IDT staff.

- The format is easier to comprehend quickly by IDT staff.

THE PATIENT'S CURRENT REVERIE

Whatever was on the patient's mind and in the patient's heart as the caregiver approached can be relevant to that person's core. What a patient is currently mulling over gives clues to her chief concerns.

- Samuel is a ten-year-old boy, *who lost his right arm in a corn picker accident two days ago and was already calmly practicing writing with his left hand in preparation for returning to school.*

- Jenny is a 52-year-old married nursing assistant, *who was speaking rapidly about her need to return to work as soon as possible as the only employed member of her family of five.*

HOW THE PATIENT RESPONDED TO THE CAREGIVER

When the patient visit is in response to a referral from another IDT member, the staff often have a special interest in how the patient related to that spiritual caregiver. Sometimes this qualifies for the special place at the end of the first sentence.

- Mr. Nexus is a 58-year-old dairy farmer, who eventually talked openly about his diminishing ability to perform the chores necessary to hold on to his farm.

- Jared is an 18-year-old varsity swimmer, *who was refreshingly forthright about his possibly letting his teammates down if his healing and rehab interfere with his contributions to the team this winter.*

Finding words for describing your impression of a patient's response to you or her current attitude benefits from developing the caregiver's own taxonomy of adverbs and adjectives that one finds useful. Suggested adverbs to start with include: guardedly, warmly, openly, critically, eagerly, gratefully, tearfully, and suspiciously. Adjectives include: forthright, chatty, grumpy, taciturn, sullen, feisty, sad, and aggravated.

RECENT FAMILY HAPPENINGS, ATTITUDES, MUSINGS, OR CONFLICTS

Personal and interpersonal information about what is happening with key family members regarding the patient's situation can sometimes help clinicians make decisions about how to approach them with new information or serious medical decisions that need to be made.

- I saw Serena, referred by nursing as a 31-year-old single female, *currently in a bit of conflict with two of her brothers about her pondering whether or not to discontinue dialysis.*

- When I dropped in on this 38-year-old mother of three, *she was near tears over the disappointment over her youngest (14-year-old) girl's refusal to come to see her because of a disagreement that the patient sees as minor.*

A descriptive paragraph

A phenomenologically oriented chart note format follows the first sentence with a succinct descriptive or narrative paragraph. Any of the content of the first sentences listed in the previous section can be used in this paragraph if not used there. The goal is to use the stories told by the patient to capture intuitively a description of the patient in her basic humanness, as she negotiates her present condition. Putting the sentences together paints a picture of the uniqueness of this person who may appear to be nasty, sullen, obstreperous, or non-compliant in recent behavior but holds an inherent beauty as a human being.

Only rarely is it necessary to fashion paragraphs longer than this brief one, capturing her soul to the degree possible. Brevity is of high importance. Nobody in healthcare reads long, chatty notes.

In addition to the suggested first sentence stories listed above, a few others may be considered for the remainder of the paragraph. Three highly recommended ones are:

- *A quote,* a precise quotation of something the patient said that somehow summarizes a key point about the patient. There is a difference of opinion about whether or not the spiritual caregiver's own interpretation of the patient's words ought to be added. In any case, remember that the patient has a right to read her own chart note at any time, and therefore family members may read it too.

- *Who loves this patient and who disturbs him?* It can sometimes be relevant to name or otherwise document specific people and at times even include their contact information. The human spirit of us all is constantly influenced by those who love us. Noticing signs of affection in caring conversations becomes a source of information often later relevant to healthcare decisions. Likewise, identifying people who are seriously troubling to a person while hospitalized can tip off staff members to possibly significant latent interpersonal conflicts and even protection of the patient.

- *Brief religious comments, if relevant* (minimize jargon): This is still a world with quite religious populations intermingling with highly secular ones. A majority of caregivers in some geographical regions expect all spiritual caregivers to make some comment about the religious faith and practice of any patient they visit (see Chapters 2 and 3).

PASTOR D

Introduction

I encountered D as I was going down my list of patients who had not yet been seen. I only knew her admission date, age, sex, religious preference, and a very general description of her "primary problem" before entering the room. She is an 80-year-old widow and mother of Danish ancestry, who has primarily made a living as a non-denominational pastor. Her current diagnosis was uncertain and pending, but she was in the hospital due to increasing weakness and inability to use her extremities/paralysis. She has a history of other medical problems, most notably diabetes, coronary artery disease (she also has a pacemaker), hypertension, and arthritis. None of these conditions had seemed to present new symptoms that could have contributed to her current problems. When I entered the room D was lying down peacefully on her back and the room was silent. As the conversation began I was relieved that she was receptive to the visit, but I was also surprised that her speech and demeanor did not seem to fit well with her condition. Although in a seemingly vulnerable situation she was calm and confident. She seemed to have no qualms at all about being ill or being in the hospital.

Analysis

D was happy to have a visitor and even happier to have someone who was interested in her life of faith. She described her many medical problems and the presence of God throughout her travails with these problems, including those leading up to her current visit. She is on a constant quest to find God's peace, as she sees this peace as her guiding light. I sensed that her current dramatic loss of arm and leg functioning and the loss of her husband in 2012 were items that she may need to process, since this search for peace (supernatural) may have inhibited her ability to deal with the human realities at play (natural). Through persistent prompting, she did begin to open up about both of these losses, but seemed to drift from reminiscing and processing back into a more mechanical description of her life. Thus I think she may still benefit from more processing to deal with the emotional side of her losses and also to make sure she is prepared to embrace the reality of her current condition.

Chart note

The patient is an 80-year-old widow and mother who reports experiencing progressive problems with the functioning of her extremities (possibly related to neuropathy) in addition to a long history of medical problems, including diabetes and heart problems. Despite hardly being able to walk (even with a walker) and to lift her arms, she seemed remarkably peaceful and confident, reporting no anxiety, anger, or frustration regarding her situation. For her, as a long time non-denominational pastor, God is a huge influence in her life and she fully trusts that He will see her through. She very much enjoyed talking about her faith, her vibrant family and her ministry, and she did begin to open up about the loss of her husband (2012) and of her physical capabilities with some persistence and encouragement. She may still have grief regarding these losses, and I recommend that the chaplain team follow up with her to further pursue.

Suggested improvements

D is an 80-year-old female, widowed pastor of Danish ancestry whose rather stoic demeanor melted some during this conversation. She talks easily about her solid faith in God, which sustains her now, as she has recently lost most of the use of both her arms and her legs. She does worry a bit about her future and still grieves her husband who died two years ago. She speaks with confidence and seems to be waiting quietly for further medical insight into her present condition. We prayed, and she appeared to be happily engaged in the praying. The patient's religious beliefs seem to be a major component of her life.

- *Goal*: I will encourage the chaplains and any staff members who wish to, to continue grief work with D regarding her husband's death and her possible loss adjustment counseling due to her worries that she may not regain full use of her extremities.

RATIONALE FOR SUGGESTED IMPROVEMENTS

- Reference to specifics of the patient's physical condition is unnecessary.

- Does the chaplain have a comment about the patient's progress on adjusting to the encroaching disability?

- Was there any relevant content to the prayer as disclosed by the patient?

Summarizing the salient in bullet points

Relevant information about a patient that is not included in the first sentence or the descriptive paragraph can be fashioned into two to four bullet points. Only rarely is it necessary to write more than that. Topics of bullet points that are commonly used are:

- identified spiritual needs (see Chapter 3)

- information about family members or friends who are involved in the patient's current situation

- comments about the religious background and practice and/or usefulness as resources for the resilience of the patient

- a quick summary of the spiritual care provided

- goals of care that make up a "plan" consisting of what the visiting caregiver intends to do to address any spiritual needs

- outcomes as actually observed (see Chapter 6).

The Joint Commission on Accreditation of Healthcare Organizations (JCAHO) has a specific focus on the staff's goals of care for the patient, the spiritual care provided by the caregiver to meet the goals, and on the caregiver's plan.

CHEM DEP WRECKAGE

Introduction

I walked into the room to find a man alone, lying in bed, with what appeared to be severe chemical burns on his face and mouth. He had large blisters on his tongue and lips, and was having to constantly wipe drool from his mouth with a towel because he couldn't close his mouth fully. He has short, curly hair with a salt and pepper look to it, broad shoulders, and a sad demeanor. It was pretty early in the morning when I started visiting with the patient, and this visit lasted for almost a full hour.

Analysis

I walked in and visited with a patient who is in a very low point in his life. During our hour-long conversation we talked about everything from needing God's help on the one hand to reminiscing about beating people with a baseball bat in exchange for drugs on the other. The patient was at times quite sad and even tearful, and at other times he was able to express humor about past events. I wonder how serious he is about his plan to turn his life around; from our conversation I didn't think he really had any kind of positive support system. He does have people in his life, but they appear to have a negative influence on him to the point of trapping him in this self-destructive lifestyle. I wonder if he has the opportunity or even the ability to make some positive changes in his living situation, in order to pursue sobriety as he said he wanted to.

Chart note

The patient is a 40-year-old male, who is currently on his fourth hospitalization for drug overdose. He has bad chemical burns from inhaling industrial cleaning aerosols, and is currently in a very vulnerable state in terms of his emotions. The patient expresses regret for the lifestyle he has made thus far, and is very interested in spiritual care, but claims to not be "ready just yet." The patient appears to want to take his life in a healthier direction, but does not have any sort of support system for doing so. I recommended follow-up about his desire for forgiveness with a priest based on the patient's own plans to speak with a priest on the Native American reservation where the patient lives.

Suggested improvements

The patient is a 40-year-old male member of a local Native American tribe in his fourth hospitalization for drug overdose, who talked openly with me for an hour about the many regrets of his life that he attributes largely to his chemical addiction. His vague spiritual yearnings and spoken good intentions for fashioning a better life need assessment by an addictions professional for potential motivation for treatment and its funding. He seems to be in a short window of vulnerability and pain caused by his chemical usage leading to this hospitalization that may constitute an opportunity for his acceptance of referral for addiction treatment. The patient cried while talking about his life regrets and verbalizes motivation to find a recovery lifestyle.

- *Goal*: The patient needs assessment for addiction, possibly to be followed by treatment and then Twelve Step involvement. I will urge the social worker to arrange this if possible.

- *Goal*: The patient has historical ties to Roman Catholic culture for which he nurtures sentiment, so I also referred him to a Catholic priest on the reservation for care of his massive guilt.

RATIONALE FOR SUGGESTED IMPROVEMENTS

This visit was both monumental in the patient's life and only a start to a very difficult but possible recovery life. Almost all chaplains need refined skills for addressing addiction that are not taught in CPE. Mentioning that the patient cried while talking about his regrets is a clue to an addictions counselor that a bit of Step One may have been accomplished here that can be used in treatment if resources can be found for this patient to receive it.

We have introduced answers to why spiritual perspectives should be recorded in the medical record, outlined a humanistic theory of spirituality to guide the content of spiritual care listening, identified spiritual needs common to hospitalized people, and suggested a format for spiritual care notes. The process of creating a note remains difficult to represent. However, there are some reflections that can help develop a style of doing so, consisting of consideration on who has a stake in reading the notes, and the functions involved in note construction. We turn now to some comments on that process.

5

Process

Extracting the Relevant

The effort really to see and really to represent is no idle business in face of the constant force that makes for muddlement.

HENRY JAMES (BLACKMUR 1983, P.21)

The process of creating an elegant, or even a useful, charting note includes more than identifying needs and filling in a format. Working among diverse other professionals compels a spiritual caregiver to quickly consider several points of view when charting. She will be paying attention to the well-defined practice cultures of several professional healthcare disciplines who may read her observations. She will take into consideration other key perspectives that are mostly foreign to her, such as ethics, the law, and anyone to whom she may refer a patient for another form of care. Eventually that complex process will become easier with experience as she develops her own flow of combining multiple considerations in writing a five-minute note. But learning to do so initially takes some dedicated discipline, and continuing to do so as part of a profession requires a lively spirit of persistent learning all through a career.

As we saw in Chapter 2, patient disclosure that is facilitated to run its own course *from the patient's point of view*, can be extremely complex and in content actually encompass all of life. So as we approach the computer to chart we need to sort through patient and family information, deciding what to ignore and what is salient. The data of a single conversation can be seen through at least eight essential lenses as illustrated below. Figure 5.1 illustrates the various considerations to be held in mind as a spiritual caregiver decides and writes about what is most currently relevant.

The term "consider" originated as a sailing term. It means literally to "study the stars" in navigation (Latin *cum* meaning "with" and *sidus* meaning "star"). In our context the combination means "to study something together" in order to find direction in a complex situation of shared responsibility. In a real sense the spiritual caregiver is shaping her note together with the patient and other IDT members, while remaining cognizant of the courts where the note may someday be used in legal proceedings. As a human description, a spiritual care chart note written well can be easily understood by other interested humans as it draws attention to needs of patients without any hint of moralizing, pejorative attitudes, or superfluous self-reference, and with no more than a minimum of theological jargon. Remember that note might be read by the patient five minutes after it is written, and needs to be appreciated by her and her family members as accurate, relevant, and sometimes instructive, even when its content is sad and scary.

Who are the regular and occasional readers of this note and what are the various processes involved in shaping it?

Considering the readers of chart notes

ETHICAL PERSPECTIVES: CONFIDENTIALITY
The semi-sacred tone of the word "confidentiality" has widely dissuaded chaplains from being candid, substantive, and clear in their chart notes.

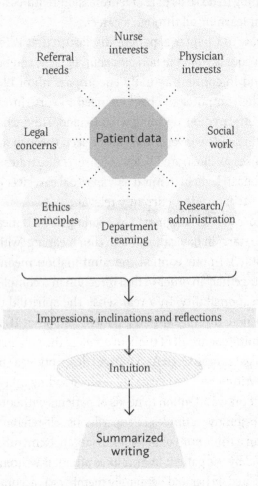

Figure 5.1 A chart note formulation process

Citing the long ecclesiastical tradition of the "seal of confession," some still erect impervious barriers to sharing patient disclosures with the IDT, in a robust guarding of their self-perceived unique specialness. Effectively, collaborative spiritual caregivers, however, transcend that misplaced hyper-reverence that often serves as rationalization for some chaplains to distance themselves from the earthy and often irreverent milieu of healthcare teams. Developing a realistic, functional, and effective use of the concept of confidentiality remains a prerequisite to establishing a professional spiritual caregiver practice.

The term "confidentiality" is derived from combining the Latin *com* meaning "with" and *fidere* meaning "to trust." Together they refer to the promotion of personal disclosure through assumed trust such as that we all feel when we approach a physician for help. The purpose of confidentiality is to foster a culture of confidence in a specific group of professional helpers who routinely share sensitive information with one another to optimize the care of patients. The staff members who are covered by that umbrella essentially agree to openly share personal information about patients and guard that data from anybody outside that team. Those outside the particular treatment unit face an institutional policy and an ethical compliance barrier to acquire that information.

When a spiritual caregiver begins to contribute to the flow of beneficial information among a specific staff, she effectively joins that team. When she commonly withholds significant patient information obtained through spiritual caring conversations, she excludes herself from full membership of that team. One does not come to belong in an IDT by somebody else allowing her in or putting her on a list of members. She joins by making actual contributions to the primary work of that team. That is why quality chart notes are so crucial to spiritual caregivers initiating themselves as full team members.

The more obvious problems with confidentiality arise when some aspects of information about patients actually do not belong in the chart. Patients have a right to the privacy of specific information that could harm their reputation forever, especially if that information is not pertinent to the work of the team. Out of sensitivity for patient preferences and respect for every patient's rights of privacy, some personal information is not only unnecessary but dissemination of it anywhere is unethical. Specifics of a patient's history of abuse, for example, and past errant and irrelevant behavior, need to be excluded from writing about patient's stories. For such long past historical behaviors as rape, combat atrocities, child abuse, sibling violence, and adolescent sexual experimentation, it is enough to generalize in reporting it, if it is relevant at all. The questions can rather be whether: 1) to share such disclosures orally with selected team members; 2) to chart them in general rather than in specific terms; or 3) to not share them at all. A patient's regrets from the past that still come to her mind accompanied by rekindled guilt benefit from "confession" but are not necessarily to be confessed or disclosed to any more than one person, the caregiver who hears them directly.

What information disclosed by a patient can and should be recorded according to principles of professional ethics, and what must be left out? Patients open up privately to hospital staff members and spiritual/ religious leaders because of their assumptions that the information will be treated with discretion. Any decisions about what portions of information regarding the human spirit belong in the medical record require brief discernment through the established windows of beneficence, non-maleficence, utility, and assessing the unique contextual factors. In short, the note writer can ask herself if what she is including in the medical record is likely to: 1) not hurt the patient in any way imaginable; 2) benefit her significantly; 3) be realistically functional for the human community; and 4) optimally fit into the complex deliberations about the patient's current medical situation.

David McCurdy (2012), as an ethicist and CPE supervisor, and others like him, have dedicated considerable work to studying and teaching about chaplain charting and the right to privacy in healthcare systems. Their perspectives on the basic principles and fine points of confidentiality in spiritual care charting should be consulted by anyone seriously interested in comprehending this subject. Spiritual caregivers' comments about the human spirits of patients are as highly sensitive as any interaction anywhere and can become difficult with their unique complexity. When any caregiver begins to comment on patients and their care, he takes on responsibility to protect that information by keeping it within the bounds of the IDT in which they work. He also agrees to divulge only what may reasonably be assumed to be in the best interest of the patient.

To be quite sure of remaining in compliance with confidentiality requirements in writing, a spiritual caregiver can generally rely on four basic principles: 1) staying conscious of putting the patient's interests first; 2) respecting some patient disclosures as sacred and distinguishing those from information that the patient would reasonably not mind being disseminated among members of that specific IDT; 3) creating all notes with such respect that they universally hold the patient in a positive light, honoring her as a fine human being at least as important as the caregiver and anyone else anywhere; and 4) informing and discussing with the patient anything he, in your best judgement, might not want in the chart. If you have any questions about him possibly wanting specific aspects of conversations left out of the chart completely, ask him or don't disclose them, except where you are bound by law to report to the authorities. The need for the latter occurs rarely but when it does it is highly important that your integrity in following these principles and the state laws is intact. As noted below, in the next section, the 50 US states differ considerably in their laws about when and how such requirements are to be made.

The basics of these concerns should be learned by chaplains and other caregivers during the early stages of their formative education. But life itself is far more complicated than principles and policies can make easy. The art of charting well, including brief relevant narratives, relies on developing the ability to describe people richly and highlight their essential goodness while continuing to abide by the ethical boundaries of healthcare culture. As with any art, continued learning along with inspiration, imagination, and willingness to learn from consultation around unpredictable moments optimize the continued growth of excellence.

LEGAL IMPLICATIONS

In addition to whether a given chart entry is ethical, there is the concern about whether it is also legal. When a chart note is brought into court it is essentially leaving the umbrella of confidentiality of that hospital unit in which it was written. The writer of that note may then be subpoenaed to testify about what she saw and heard that prompted the note. Most spiritual caregivers will never be accused of anything illegal appearing in their charting, nor asked to testify about events they record there. But it does happen. An experienced palliative care medical practitioner has told me that only twice in her career had she seen chaplain notes being involved directly in court proceedings. Both of them involved chaplains' unintentional misrepresentation. Both had used medical or psychiatric language in patient assessment as if they were competent and authorized to do so. It is likely that they merely copied such language from physician or nursing notes, or had become so familiar with that terminology that it seemed commonly accepted to use it themselves, even in the charts. It is not.

One clear bit of advice commonly learned in orientation sessions of formative spiritual care professional education is to refrain from any word that could be seen as psychiatric, even when it has come to be normalized as humorous hyperbole in common parlance. One can refer to another person's anxiety or depression in the mechanic's garage or hair salon, for example, but in the hospital as a caregiver, especially in writing, it amounts to exceeding the boundaries of one's professional role. And if a spiritual caregiver focuses her chart note content on what in her common sense opinion is best for that patient, there is little danger she will be breaking the law. A bit of self-excitement when charting dramatic events is the enemy, quickly resulting in over-reaching one's established role as an institutional caregiver.

Another rare but crucial question of what does not belong in chart notes is the discernment about mandatory reporting of such issues of child and elder abuse or neglect. Chaplains in most states will be required to report patient mentions of child abuse.[1] But the reporting should not be done in the medical record. States clearly

---

1   It is the responsibility of any caregiver to know whether she is a mandatory reporter of child abuse and neglect by the laws of the state in which she practices. Getting oneself clear on this obligation is essential for spiritual caregivers. It is wise to make a personal commitment to report any child abuse or neglect that one becomes aware of, and informing the source if it is a patient that you will need to do so. This is true whether the caregiver is considered to be clergy in a state that maintains special regulations for clergy or not. In addition, some students may be obliged to report as part of an obligation from another professional role she holds such as a nurse, teacher, or child care worker, even if she is not considered by law to be clergy.

require specific processes for the reporting, and that action is best done in conjunction with other IDT caregivers in consultation. There are legal implications as to whether or not a spiritual caregiver is a mandatory reporter in any given state. These include differences by state in who a mandatory reporter is and whether or not a chaplain or chaplain student is considered to be clergy. But in any case, the process of reporting does not include doing so in the medical record (see Sullivan 2014).

SUSPECTED DOMESTIC VIOLENCE[2]

A spiritual caregiver visits with a patient who appears to IDT members to have been bruised by being hit. Nobody has written anything in the chart that there are suspicions that the person who hit her lives with her. In conversation with a chaplain, however, she softly defends for a while but eventually acknowledges that her husband does slap her around from time to time when she "loses control of her mouth." The patient has forbidden the chaplain to tell anybody, because her husband will find out and she'll have to take the dire physical consequences. What does the caregiver write in the chart about this and what does she do then?

This is actually not a rare scenario. The woman needs help that she is initially refusing to accept. The caregiver is not generally mandated by law to disclose the abuse to authorities. Can she record something in the chart and then work with the woman on accepting help from a women's shelter? If so, what can she write? The chaplain's heart cannot simply pass this by. Yet her mind struggles as to how to proceed.

SOME SUGGESTIONS

- Do nothing until consulting with other clinical caregivers responsible for the woman's care.

2   These examples are composites of real reports that have been anonymized.

- Write in the chart something like: This is a 43-year-old married woman who cried as she talked about being admitted to the ER for bruises and possible internal injuries from a physical attack. She reports feeling trapped but initially refused counseling assistance.

- *Goal*: As patient calms and further regains her best thinking, continue to engage her about an appropriate referral.

- *Goal*: Inform patient about the state law regarding domestic violence.

- I listened thoroughly and referred the patient to an ER social worker for this approach.

- Domestic violence is against the law, but there is no obligation for a chaplain to report it in the medical record. His obligation is to collaborate with IDT members in the difficult care needed.

ELDER NEGLECT

In visiting with an 80-year-old partially disabled woman in a gerontology hospital unit, a chaplain hears her say in tears that she becomes intensely lonely when her 27-year-old grandson doesn't attend to her for days at a time. She can't always feed and bathe herself and has no other family in the area. What might the chaplain write in the medical record and what can he do after that?

- First consult with a unit caregiver, nurse and/or social worker, disclosing the alleged neglect and deciding together what to do next.

- Discern whether or not the patient is a credible reporter of her own experience. Your further questions about unrelated topics such as her medical condition, asking her to "teach back" what she has learned about it, may offer hints as to both her decisional capacity and her mental competence. This project will likely include consultation or referral.

- Report the interaction to the proper authorities designated by state law.

- Consider contacting the grandson or another family member if one can be found. Is there any legal or otherwise assigned obligation for the grandson to care for his grandmother? Has he been designated as the one person responsible to do so, as she implies?

Chart note

Nellie is an 80-year-old Caucasian woman who cries when telling about her home situation and the loneliness and neglect it causes her. I contacted nursing and the medical social worker regarding further assistance for the patient.

- *Goal*: Ascertain contact information for the patient's grandson and suggest the social worker engage him about the allegations— or do it yourself.

- *Goal*: Assist the social worker, if necessary, to ascertain whether the grandson needs assistance with his care of this patient and possibly arrange for that help.

- *Goal*: Report the possible elder neglect to the state authorities.

- *Goal*: Continue supportive care of the patient while hospitalized.

Elders are vulnerable adults in many states. Abuse or neglect of them is against the law for designated caregivers and must be reported by anyone becoming aware of it. The government and volunteer services for abuse and neglect in most locations remain patchy and coordination among those responsible is often inefficient. Still, this woman needs physical care and lack of it is also a pressing spiritual need. Doing what is required by law and whatever else is possible to meet these needs is a moral and ethical obligation of a spiritual caregiver even when any legal responsibilities have been met.

The immediate interdisciplinary context

It is widely assumed by chaplains that only a few IDT members at their healthcare facility read their notes seriously. In a 2015 quality improvement study at a large urban medical center with a solid reputation, however, CPE residents used a simple, locally designed survey instrument to test that assumption for their facility (see Appendix for the full study report). The study was too small to qualify as professional research and a request to expand it to make it qualify was finally rejected by the chief executive officer. She wisely noted that it would not be a positive precedent to elicit evaluative comments about one discipline from other disciplines. The implications of having nurses evaluate chart notes of doctors, for example, was daunting. The study that was conducted, however, largely disputed the assumptions about IDT members not reading chart notes written about spiritual care in that facility.

The survey was distributed at random to IDT members on hospital units not served by the distributing residents to minimize sympathetic responses. The instrument elicited answers to five questions:

1. How often do you seek spiritual care medical record notes for insight into understanding your patients?

2. How often do you read a spiritual care note when you see one?

3. In what percentage do you find spiritual care notes to be understandable?

4. In what percentage do you find spiritual care notes to be substantive?

5. In what percentage do you find spiritual care notes to be useful?

The results of this informal study are illustrated below.

Table 5.1 IDT members who seek spiritual care chart notes

	n	Most of the time	Often	Hardly ever	Never
Registered nurses	86	12 14.0%	32 37.2%	34 39.5%	8 9.3%
Medical doctors	12	0 0.0%	4 33.3%	7 58.3%	1 8.3%
Other	18	2 11.1%	2 11.1%	10 55.6%	4 22.2%
Total	116	14 12.0%	38 32.8%	51 44.0%	13 10.3%

Table 5.2 IDT members who read spiritual care notes when they see one

	n	Most of the time	Often	Hardly ever	Never
Registered nurses	86	27 31.4%	33 28.4%	20 23.3%	6 7.0%
Medical doctors	12	2 16.7%	5 41.7%	4 33.3%	1 8.3%
Other	18	2 11.0%	7 38.9%	5 27.8%	4 22.2%
Total	116	31 26.7%	45 39.0%	29 25.0%	11 9.5%

Spiritual care notes, on a 1–10 scale, were found to be:

- understandable—average rating, all, 8.1

- substantive—average rating, all, 7.2

- useful—average rating, all, 7.3.

Clearly there were too few respondents to confirm IDT responses as accurate with any research confidence. However, it remains interesting to note that at that world-class medical center in which chaplains are quite well-integrated into systems of care, the results showed that:

- 60 percent of nurses often or most of the time read a spiritual care note when they see one.

- About 45 percent of IDT respondents either most of the time or often seek available chart notes to better understand their patients, and about 55 percent hardly ever or never do.

- About 65 percent of IDT respondents either most of the time or often read a spiritual care note when they see one in the chart, while 35 percent hardly ever or never do.

- The average rating of IDT members for the quality of chaplain notes (understandable 8.1, substantive 7.3, and useful 7.2, on a 1–10 scale) is encouraging.

Overall, the study suggests that a number of clinicians are already interested in what chaplains write in the chart and it can be assumed that more would read them if spiritual care chart notes improved to better fit the mindset and daily practice patterns of clinicians' work. The spaces provided for narrative comments in electronic medical records (EMRs) could be better used by spiritual caregivers interested in communicating clearly with IDTs.

The study hypothesized that *narrative* charts would be read more often and usefully than the boxes and lines currently being emphasized by research and efficiency-minded facilities. That hypothesis could not be studied comprehensively at that time (2014).

WHAT NURSES WANT TO KNOW ABOUT A PATIENT'S HUMAN SPIRIT

Care of the human spirit has been an integral part of nursing since its professionalized beginnings with Florence Nightingale. Even before that, from ancient times, nurses have always been moved by the human spirit's suffering, confusion, and ignorance of what is best for its bodily self-care. Currently, however, nurses are plagued by daunting responsibilities from the volume of patient care, administrative structures, and regulatory demands. Providing any kind of spiritual care as a nurse in most positions is almost always out of the question.

But that spark of dedication to the human spirit continues to nudge nurses' souls underneath their daily overwork.

Nurses vary considerably in their interest in praying with their patients and in the religiosity of their patients in general. But describing the state of the human spirit of patients and commenting about it among themselves is a natural part of nursing practice. Nurses typically reflect on and converse with one another—"How is Mrs. Smith doing?"—referring to more than patients' physical state. Deepening their answers to that question using the concepts in this book could be a step ahead for some nurses and for the profession as a whole. Those nurses who nurture a natural curiosity about the inner workings of the hearts and minds of patients are fostering a humanistic practice of caring and its greater level of career satisfaction.

A spiritual caregiver's note that is brief, pointed, a narrative for humanness, and relevant to the patient's condition will be read by a majority of nurses when they see it in the medical record. Nurses pay attention to patient needs for improving their human spirits and for the availability of whatever and whoever is likely to support this. They want to know what they can about immediate needs for physical comfort, including patient disclosures about pain levels. Include in chart notes what you know about significant and relevant family issues. For nurses' interest, also consider charting about patient attitudes about their medical condition, treatment, and relationships with staff members. When pointedly and accurately summarized, these help nurses fill their care-full curiosity.

WHAT PHYSICIANS MIGHT VALUE ABOUT SPIRITUAL CARE

Physicians are generally interested in what spiritual caregivers can make clear regarding a patient's attitudes about his health situation and treatment. Negative patient satisfaction scores are most often based on those attitudes left unaddressed, because they were not perceived by IDT members. While spiritual care chart notes are not written only for physicians, aiming them at physicians enhances their usefulness for everyone involved.

Physicians cannot be stereotyped any more than any other professional, ethnic, or social group. But the process of becoming an MD does seem to place doctors in specific roles that are best understood only by one another. They differ widely in their interest in spiritual care comments in their practice, often depending on the acuity of a given patient. Medical schools are evolving to include much more attention to emotional connection, interpersonal communication, and cognizance of the "patient experience." However, there is still a considerable distance to go along the path of actual integrated medicine as a realistic expectation of patients. When patient satisfaction is determined by phone calls to discharged patients with questions that are often not seen by medical practitioners as relevant to medical practice, the distance widens between medical practitioners and society, a most unfortunate eventuality. The excessive expectations that society has of physicians, who are also incessantly coerced by regulatory and insurance agreements, administrative harshness, and the demands of research data collection, combine to push today's physicians to far less satisfying lives than they had hoped for when entering medical school.

Still, physicians deeply interested in helping people and making a contribution to the human community at least glance at what spiritual caregivers are trying to do. If they find disappointment there, they mostly ignore spiritual care notes from that spiritual caregiver altogether. If they find assistance in helping patients human to human, they vibrate towards that service and value chaplaincy. In short, they value spiritual caregiving that is practical, knowledgeable, and communicated in common terms.

Physicians can generally become interested in spiritual care notes when one note makes sense to the care of a specific patient. Such a note is brief, to the point, readable, human, astute about that patient's current predicament, and focused on the inner workings of that person's core. Patient attitudes toward their condition, their treatment, their progress, and their future are of particular interest to doctors. Doctors want help with the personal and interpersonal aspects of care but rarely articulate that and are not accustomed to validating it when they see it. It is not their job to tell spiritual caregivers how to do their job. If those caregivers do not seem to be offering anything relevant to patients, doctors generally ignore them, usually staying tolerant and polite but internally shaking their heads as they walk away.

PARTNERING WITH SOCIAL WORKERS

Social workers, like most healthcare professionals, are variously trained. Influenced by many other professional fields, they cluster in two groups as either medical or psychiatric social workers. Founded over time in the late 19th century to improve living conditions of poor populations, they emphasized practical assistance, differing from the more philosophical and religious approach of pastors. They became professionalized about the same time chaplaincy transformed from highly religious towards more clinical in the mid-1920s. Medical social work had its origin to a great extent in Boston about the same time and place that clinical pastoral education began injecting clinical perspectives into institutional pastoral care (Dulmus and Sowers 2012).[3]

Today medical social workers emphasize helping patients make connections to various forms of care after hospital discharge. Psychiatric social workers, on the other hand, concentrate in mental health programs and private practice therapy. Medical social workers work to improve patients' access to groups and communities that can assist them with medical and living difficulties. They particularly serve more disadvantaged people who do not as easily find and make use of social services and specialty treatment programs. They are likely to value spiritual caregivers for their keen descriptions of people and sometimes for their knowledge of religious values and practices. If they use the perspectives of religion and spirituality in their practices, they tend to see them as social support, basic life guidance, healthy behavioral frameworks, and calming self-care routines.

The broad notion of spirituality used in this book unsettles some social workers who see chaplains, for example, as overstepping their

---

3   Social workers eventually organized themselves into the American Association of Social Workers in 1921.

limits in areas such as addictions, mental illness, hostility, and family conflict. Often they are right. But an alternative view is also cogent. Social workers actually practice spiritual care by this book's broader definition, only wisely ignoring or minimizing the value of its religious component. In any case there is often a subtle competitiveness between social workers and spiritual caregivers in any given institution. That competition eventuality dissolves in the shared responsibility of actual care from a humanistic focus on specific individuals. Most all social workers seem to value spiritual care chart notes that are realistically descriptive.

SPIRITUAL CARE TEAM INTERESTS

Hospital chaplain departments vary in their commitment to collaborating among themselves for comprehensive care of widely diverse patient populations and families. Those chaplains who value such sharing of responsibility for the institution would want to formulate at least informal policies about what to chart in order to pass cases to another chaplain shift or to a specific colleague chaplain, and to maintain a record of referrals made to other forms of care. It is common to create logs separate from the medical record used exclusively by chaplains for their collaborative work. Actual chart notes with colleagues in mind typically include information congruent with the chart note format described in Chapter 4. They may also include phone or pager numbers of family members and contact information of other individuals they know are highly interested in a given case.

ADMINISTRATIVE OVERSIGHT

Administration has a few primary interests in spiritual caregivers' work and also some pertinent questions about their institutional chaplains. For example, "Do they make public relations better, with pleasing behavior, or worse, with glaring and deeply troubling mistakes?" "Do they improve patient satisfaction scores?" And "What do chaplains do that adds value to healthcare outcomes?" Certainly there are administrators who support spiritual care teams because they believe that the broadly understood spiritual aspect of human beings contributes to healthcare outcomes and to human resilience. And there are also those who do so because it is the humane thing to do. Still others do so for political, image management reasons. There are still many who do not support spiritual care at all, largely because it smacks of religion that has previously become distasteful or peripheral to the lives of those particular administrators.

In general, a hospital administrator will not inspect spiritual care programs unless they cause problems, and some of those problems stem from inappropriate chart notes that find their way into ethics committees and the courts. However, there is some movement among administrative leaders in championing, endorsing, or at least permitting research studies that help them analyze the performance of chaplains. That interest actually resulted in spiritual care charting formats that are designed with checking boxes and filling lines to optimize the ease of collecting data. Many administrators and managers, both inside and outside the field of clinical chaplaincy, settle for numbers about something that seems to point to quality rather than any inspection of chaplain chart notes as depictions of depth of care for the human spirit. As spiritual caregivers improve the actual usefulness of their chart notes, anecdotal evidence will increasingly be added to the already substantial evidence basis for appreciating the value of spiritual care.

PREPARATION FOR REFERRALS

Professionals such as psychologists, social workers, and various therapists with access to the medical record will often be briefed by phone or text on the essential information for them to grasp the reason for the referral. But in addition, brief, official comments on the state of the human spirit of the person being referred can alert the referent to intricacies of the patient situation that are not included in the phone referral. While the text or phone call conveys highly confidential unique detail, the stories in the chart note may provide broader human situational context and recent event information. A person receiving a referral can read several chart notes before seeing the patient and put together a process of the reason for referral over time.

Spiritual caregivers making a referral of a hospital patient are also alerting IDT members of the acuity perceived by that note writer regarding a patient issue that may be only vaguely noticed, or not perceived at all by the IDT as a whole. Including the reason for referral clearly, in common terms, in a chart note comprehensively alerts the entire staff that a substantive patient issue is being addressed. That has value even if the referral is to a person from outside the hospital to a resource who does not have access to the medical record, such as a pastor, counselor or Twelve Step program sponsor. It helps IDT members know how to brief the person receiving the referral when she arrives.

Distilling the note content

IMPRESSIONS, REFLECTIONS, AND INCLINATIONS

A young female chaplain student was attending staff meetings in her assigned palliative care residency setting, remaining silent and observing. A physician asked her at one point why she was so quiet in the meetings. She explained that she was observing to keep learning about the service and that particular modality. He kindly told her that her job there was to tell the other staff members what she has learned about the inner world of the patients. He not only included her with the word "other" staff members, but validated her humanity and the value of her sharing her experiences of what the patients were thinking, feeling, and saying as well as fearing, questioning, yearning for, and grieving. Aware that she knew almost nothing about the process and the various roles of the different disciplines gathered there, he wanted her impressions.

Impressions are the aspects of patient conversations that make a significant imprint on the listener. They constitute what is most easily remembered. Even as one is only beginning to learn to listen personally and care-fully, some words, topics, and emotions stand out among what one learns from a single conversation with a patient. Learning what impressions may be relevant to a given IDT takes time, experience, and astute observation. It also takes trial and error. One needs to ready oneself for critique. That is often the only way to learn a skill so complex and new.

Reflections can carry more weight than impressions. They are "bendings" of the mind (Latin *reflectere*—to bend again), the fruit of mulling something over to fit sensate observations into some cognitive shape. The word actually means "to re-bend," to roll something around in the mind to find a different "bending," one that is insightful, communicative, to the point, and in this case useful to others. Reflections proceed from engaging the mind. They can happen even as one is writing down basic information, summarized stories, and impressions. Without reflection by the writer, chart entry impressions can be summarily inane, extraneous, overgeneralized, and easy to ignore. Or they can easily become irrelevant, innocuous, pedantic, and even annoying.

One's *inclinations* are "leanings," actions a listener feels like performing, what one naturally wants to do in response to what one hears and sees. They are mostly to be left inside the caregiver, not communicated to others but only used to inform yourself about how the person is affecting you. They can point to memories of other people you have previously met, impulses to embrace, leave, correct, or overindulge the storyteller. Only occasionally can they be useful in charts, to illustrate a tendency that many people may share upon meeting that person and not be able to articulate. "Seeing his pathetic, unkempt condition I just felt like wanting to get him a shower, a shave, and a clean sleep for the night," for example.

Awareness of one's own impressions, reflections, and inclinations generally improves patient descriptions towards more useful representations of the humanity of patients and family members. Much of clinical pastoral education is intended to improve that awareness, as well as cognizance of the attitudes, values, and assumptions that blur or distort their clarity in a caregiver's mind. Earthy IDT members and other spiritual caregivers naturally value them when they are well processed before or in the process of chart note writing. Disclosing them also subtly reminds chart readers that we don't fully control our responses to patients. At best we merely observe those automatic reactions in ourselves, sort them for relevance, and consider writing about them.

IDENTIFYING ISSUES AND NEEDS

The four axes of spiritual needs described in Chapter 3 serve as one framework for identifying common spiritual needs for charting. CPE students using this assessment framework often carry the presentation of the four axes shown in Figure 5.2 with them for reference for as long as it takes to incorporate it easily from memory into their daily patient care work. In facilities that still use boxes to be checked and lines to be filled, the needs summary can be used in addition to those factual assessments by injecting narratives about needs into the spaces that major EMR software generally allows.

The difference between the terms *needs* and *issues*, as used here is that needs are more specific and refer to the pain or discomfort they cause. An issue may cause several needs and tends to emphasize what's amiss inside the person that he may be somewhat responsible to address and improve. An issue is an ordinary or crisis complex of several factors, including a person's own makeup, her choices, her conflicts with other people, and uncontrollable events that cause discomfort or pain and threaten to sabotage her happiness. It is a difficulty in living that the person may be perpetuating, such as a negative attitude about specific aspects of life, a habit of relating that tends to ruin the joy of relationships, or a series of rigid beliefs that deter or inhibit the process of maturing into the adult ability to live with ambiguities and limitations. Perfectionism, compulsions, overt racism, and grudges or resentments are examples of issues. They also may be short lived however, specific to the present situation, such as a disagreement over something that seems unjust, an overreaction to being slighted, or a misunderstanding of a basic limitation of life as found vividly in difficult medical ethics decisions. A nuance of the term issue is that the person with it could likely assuage it, at least partially, if he chose to do so.

Emotional support

1. Trauma shock – Need for support in the temporary debilitation of crisis events

2. Expressing – Need to talk and express feelings

3. Fear and anxiety – Need to reduce fright

4. Anger, hostility and resentment – Need to manage anger

5. Sadness, discouragement, despair – Need for sharing disappointing events

6. Deep hurt – Need for understanding events of perceived mistreatment

7. Empowerment – Need to identify and bolster normal or new patterns of coping

Major loss

8. Current grief – Major grief anticipated or within previous 48 hours

9. Prior grief – Major past grief being currently grieved

10. Dying – Dealing with goodbyes of the dying process

11. Life adjustment – Transforming after a major change in function or appearance

12. Estrangement – Reuniting with disconnected loved ones

Religious/spiritual practice needs

13. Religious support – Need to feel the presence of positive transcendence

14. Spiritual validation – Need to share unique ways one nurtures one's human spirit

15. Spiritual counseling – Need to discuss religious, questions, issues or wounds

16. Relief from regrets – Need for relief from guilt or shame

17. Religious/spiritual instruction – Need to learn spiritual self-care modalities

Referral needs

18. Medical ethics confusion – Need to understand or discuss treatment outcome concerns

19. Mental health/addictions – Need to explore concerns about mental health or alcohol/mood-altering chemical use

20. Love life pain – Need for listening, advice, or referral about one's love life

21. Advocacy – Need for support in finding needed care

22. Family conflict – Need for facilitation of conflict among family members

Figure 5.2 Needs summary

A need, on the other hand, tends to be more specific. Spiritual needs, as described in Chapter 3, can be identified by close observation and conversation, are generally not met totally, and can often be assuaged by caring interventions. Figure 5.2 illustrates briefly the 22 spiritual needs in common terms easily recognized in patient conversations.

QUOTES TO CLINCH IMPRESSIONS

Selecting a quote from all that a patient said during a spiritual care conversation may be the best way to convey the state of that person's spirit as the caregiver encountered it. Frequently, as a caregiver walks away from a patient interaction, a specific statement made by that person stays with the listener. Alertness to that enduring quality can, upon reflection, identify the best quote for that note. It doesn't take long. It won't extend the length of a caregiver's day. And it can clinch a salient point or impression.

Quotes need to be put in quotation marks and stated in the exact words in which they were said. They ought never to contain disparaging remarks about anybody, especially IDT members, spiritual care colleagues, or the facility itself. Those remarks belong somewhere other than in the medical record, if there is good reason to communicate them at all. Still, using quotes of patient concerns crisply identifies a patient's own inner experience for IDT members, highlights the uniqueness of that person, and ties into the humanness of staff and patients alike.

PATIENT HOPES

Palliative care services have discovered that a primary direction to take with people who are suffering with serious and possibly fatal conditions is the actual hopes of that person in their current human state. Patients are often not aware of their primary hopes as one might expect them to be. But as the depth of their medical situation descends upon their reflections, hopes emerge in their minds that may be blurted out to anybody nearby. Sometimes that will be a spiritual caregiver as the patient discusses serious medical specifics. As the conversation expands on what the implications are, a given person's hopes for the future can become a major aspect of quality palliative and even general hospital care. When a patient mentions her hopes for future accomplishments or experiences tomorrow or later this year, she is creating what is now commonly called a "bucket list." It humanizes an IDT to have those hopes and discussions about a patient included in a spiritual care chart note.

Conversations with patients in whom there is an indication of a drinking problem exemplify the intricacy of focus on patient hopes. The vague spiritual yearnings characteristic of mid-stage and late-stage chemically dependent people is actually part of the unconscious denial system that shields a person from feeling the massive guilt and fear that hides within. The rosiness, victimhood, or hostility apparent in the addicted person's attitude is far more resilient than straight people ever imagine. Engaging patient hopes will usually net nothing useful. It only indulges or bounces off the fantasies that cover the terrible negative emotions that pervade the insides, of which the person, unbelievably, is mostly unaware. What can offer a bit of hope is a caregiver's persistently gentle but firm focus on the *concerns* that person has about his drug usage. One can almost never see these from the outside, except briefly, at moments of vulnerability like during hospitalization.

Learning to focus doggedly on the patient's own concerns about her usage is key and very difficult. Chaplains, like family members, tend to veer off into their own concerns or remind the patient (for the 117th time) of what they are doing to their families and their own bodies. Such moralizing always quickly fails. Describing the invaluable skills needed is outside the scope of this book. Recording summaries of such conversations, however, by those who have the skills, makes a major contribution to patients during the window of vulnerability that hospitalization grants them. It also contributes to the learning of IDT members, albeit only case by case.

PATIENTS' RELATIONSHIPS WITH THEIR CAREGIVERS

A colleague clinical supervisor of mine worked as a chaplain and chaplain educator in the same hospital for 41 years. He served on its governing board and enjoyed unusually solid relationships with administrators as they came and went, many physicians, and hundreds of nurses. Still an inveterate jogger at 66, he recognized near the end of his daily run one day that a massive fatigue was quickly descending upon him. Nearing his house he urged his wife to drive him to the emergency department of his hospital. His spleen ruptured on the way, and in the diagnosis physicians discovered that he had a sarcoma growing on his liver. He was partially conscious during the crisis care and intensive care that followed, lasting over a week and leading to chemotherapy. In the intensive care unit process he became the subject of the care of many of the clinical caregivers he had known for so long. Through the partial fog of his traumatic response, he made many observations of what their care felt like, some that surprised and mostly disappointed him.

He later called the new and brilliant clarity he experienced "liminal space." Nearly dying and a week in intensive care imposed on him a radical clarity as he saw and felt far more vividly the attitudes caregivers carried about their jobs and their relationship with him.[4] Some of the chaplains he had trained and who had become colleagues seemed to be distracted by his celebrity and the prospects of what might now happen to the department he had shaped and managed for decades. He sensed the brusque jerkiness of some hands on him that felt slightly angry and almost abusive. He noticed the curt and annoyed tone of a diagnosing physician who first disclosed the cancer to him, the hostile feel of a man who extubated him, and the incredible expectations of one nurse that he apply a soothing cream himself—to his back. He recognized those visitors who lingered beyond the time it felt to him to be enough, for whatever reason. He became painfully beleaguered by most touches being ones that caused pain, however necessary, in various areas of his body, often without comment. And then he could not believe the level of solace he received from ten minutes of gentle care in massage by a single nurse. He died ten days later.

The collaborative project we call healing flourishes to a great extent in the relationships between patients and their caregivers. In the heat

---

4   This series of events occurred similarly to those of Jill Bolte Taylor, the Harvard Neurorology professor (see Bolte Taylor 2009).

of crisis care, clinicians sometimes forget the effect their attitudes are having on a patient personally. Sometimes unapologetic harshness is necessary in those situations, for immediacy and efficiency. But it is possible to continue remembering that the patient is aware of unkind interactions that can be enormously discouraging. Words of connection and gentle touches can feel strikingly caring.

It is noted by practicing physicians that in emergency departments and other critical care situations it can be folly for clinicians to invest too much in pleasing patients rather than giving them what solid medical practice indicates they clearly need. The intricacies of palliative care conversations succeed because teasing out the difference between what people want, what they need, and what is medically now possible in their condition, remains a fragile art. In any case, however, the relationship between a patient and her caregivers can facilitate personal healing and sometimes physical progress as well.

It can be a great temptation for a spiritual caregiver to chart patient negative comments about a staff member. Documenting such comments in writing is never a good idea. Complaints by patients are common, as one would expect of people suffering and impatient for relief. Disparaging the institutional food is a perennial practice and even seen as a sign that some seriously ill patients are getting better. But any comment a spiritual caregiver hears from a patient about her current caregivers should be weighed as to its relevance to the treatment situation. Never does a specific negative comment about a particular caregiver belong in the medical record. Recount it face to face but only if your judgement discerns that it may do some good.

The most effective relationship for a spiritual caregiver to comment on, however, is the one between the patient and herself. How the caregiver saw the patient relating to her can assure IDT members that someone is effectively addressing spiritual needs—or not. It is essential, of course, that the ongoing relationship with IDT members has convinced them that your comments are accurate and not merely image management for yourself. The chief task of an IDT regarding spiritual care is to provide new attachment experiences to people isolated to some degree by their illness, injury, or condition. The quality of the patient's relationship with her spiritual caregiver can be key to that process of reconnecting with the rest of humanity in a personally healing process.

Assessing acuity

Relevance is one thing. Acuity is another. Most patients, for example, would acknowledge some level of apprehension about their condition, treatment, or prognosis. But fear burgeoning into terror powerful enough to put a stop to scheduled surgery is another level of acuity of spiritual need. While there is no definite measure of acuity in disturbances of the human spirit, there are indicators that trigger entering a given issue disclosed by a patient into the medical record.

- *The tone of a patient's manner of speaking*, especially if it is a change from the tone when talking about previous topics, prompts a careful listen about why. Serious, somber, earnest tones; fearful, aggravated, despondent ones; or low pitches along with the bowed head of shame all warrant a closer look at what is emerging from beneath social conversational overtones.

- *Hints of alarm inside the spiritual caregiver herself* as she listens to a patient may indicate that what the patient is saying is more serious than the tone of the patient's voice. Of course, that alarm might also be an aspect of the caregiver's own issues being lit up by hearing that issue in the patient. Still, the caregiver's emotional reactions to the patient provide some of the best indications of what the patient is experiencing emotionally.

- *Referral by a medical or other healthcare professional* ought to alert one to pursue the reason for the referral, even before engaging the patient. Most every referral, or even a suggestion by a nurse about who to visit first on a given unit on a given day, warrants exploration of what are the more serious inner processes going on in this patient that may be disturbing enough for the spiritual caregiver to communicate to the team.

- *Tears* generally convey a level of acuity that is worth recording. While some tears can be manipulative, still most are not, but rather indications of soulfulness. Noting in the chart what the patient was saying while crying suggests both the seriousness of the concern and identifies its content.

- *Family member or friend* questions, requests, and urgently toned information can indicate that an issue may be serious. What they mention indicates something of their own issues but may well also show astute understanding of the patient's primary concerns.

- *Immediacy* or newness of an issue can compel a spiritual caregiver to pass on information in the chart, such as rising physical or emotional pain, recent grief situations, or a patient's current informational confusion.

The use of intuition (as distinct from guessing, embellishing and confabulation)

Mastery of the use of intuition is never complete. Like the wind it always flows freely, unpredictably, and cannot be prodded. Intuition is basically putting together bits of sensation in an uncanny way to show an overall picture of what transpired in a patient contact. Suddenly seeing the forest of the patient's current place in life made up of the trees of various observations and disclosures always remains an art. A caregiver's intuitive impressions can be perilous to record since serious error in the medical record is embarrassing, can be team-confusing, perhaps personally damaging, and can find its way into court. On the other hand, sharp intuitive grasps of any human being's current state of soul can also be the heart of caregiving relationships. Letting yourself doff the habit of analysis for a moment, and letting yourself know what you already know in some unfathomable way underneath, always remains elusive and a skill worth improving.

Using intuition includes paying attention to metaphor in patient disclosures. Patients often, and maybe always, unconsciously reveal affective inner sensations and convictions they cannot make conscious. Such revelations can be put together by an intuitive listener to the benefit of better understanding that person's current state of spirit. Remaining too certain about what you already think you know about a person sabotages this intuitive project. Richard Powers said in an interview, "Only inhabiting another's story can deliver us from certainty." And "...shared stories are the only way anyone has for escaping the straightjacket of self."[5]

Barriers to using one's intuition can also be rampant in a given caregiver, however. Guessing about the future course of a patient's condition or progress of a spiritual issue is generally too risky to hazard and has no place in the chart. Learning to catch oneself at a nagging recurrent habit of needing to "show how much you know" is begun in clinical pastoral education but optimally needs ongoing clinical supervision or active consultation to keep curbed. Embellishment, hyperbole, and even confabulation in some instances, are not intuition and are more obnoxious than helpful. An ongoing arena for processing chart notes with peers in a facilitated group context takes courage to engage in regularly. But over the lifetime of a career such consistent consultation tends to create great spiritual clinicians who observe accurately and communicate quite effectively to members of other disciplines (see the Epilogue).

---

5   Interview with Richard Powers in The Believer, February 2007. Available at www. believermag.com/issues/200702/?read=interview_powers, accessed June 19, 2016.

FRANCINE

Introduction

The patient B is a 50-year-old Catholic woman who has end-stage liver cancer. Her chart also indicated that she was depressed and had high anxiety. She was in a lot of pain and had great difficulty finding a comfortable position. She did not have sufficient strength to push herself to sit up: she held on to the side of the bed or my hand to do so. Her speeches were punctuated by "ah...euh...ah..." and grimaces when she made the slightest effort to move. Several times during the visit, she had to stop talking, adjust her position, concentrate, and then burp. She said that it was a new development; it started that day.

B began living in the US at 17. She had no family in the US; a brother comes to this country frequently for his work. Her hospital room is devoid of anything that would hint at relationships. She did not appear to have a strong affinity with the church.

I visited B many times. After an IDT round, the social worker (SW) and I discussed who we were going to see. I told her that B was on my "to visit" list; she had the same. We agreed that she would visit B that day and I would visit the following day. I was therefore surprised to receive a page late that afternoon from the SW asking me to visit. She said B was sad and lonely and wanted to see me. I responded to the page even though it was close to the end of my shift.

B was asleep, lying on her side, one arm resting lightly on the side of her forehead. Her brows were knitted, and her expression was one of an uneasy sleep. I called out her name softly and waited; she opened her eyes, slowly; she looked uncertainly at me, as if she could not remember where she was or maybe trying to figure out who I was. I introduced myself and mentioned the SW who met with her earlier that day. She motioned for me to sit and she groaned as she tried to pull herself up.

Analysis

The first visit was at the expressed request of the patient; she talked slowly, appeared reticent about providing much personal information. The interaction in the first visit was not continuous, there were many silent moments, or moments when the only thing happening was the patient trying to find a comfortable position accompanied by her distress and frustration at not finding one, and her moans. The chaplain felt helpless at not being able to help the patient through her pain and felt frustrated, in fact a little angry, that requests for assistance for the patient went unmet. The patient's reticence seemed to lift in the course of the visit, though her engagement was circumscribed by her pain.

Chart note

- Visit yesterday in response to request by SW B2. Patient is struggling with sense of isolation and pain.

- Patient was laying on her side, facing the wall, completely covered, eyes closed. Responded to my greetings, appeared drawn, and very low energy. Reported being in great physical discomfort ("aching all over") and feeling weak; had difficulty pulling herself to sitting position; stopped speaking several times in the course of the visit to find a position that will enable her to burp; the need to concentrate to burp was a new development, she said.

- Patient was slow to engage in meeting; but going at her pace (expressed a dislike for loud noise or voices) seemed to have helped build trust, enabling her to reflect on various aspects of her life.

- Patient is from Kuwait; does not have much family support here, except for a brother named Samuel who lives in Kuwait.

- Chaplain offered gentle guidance to help patient who seemed to be feeling very low. She professed, "I don't have a happy place." We explored color association...hers is red, which she associated with fire, music, dance, and particularly belly dancing and flamenco, and chic; she managed a spontaneous smile and nodded when I said, "That's your happy place."

- Subsequent to meeting, I apprised her nurse, who said that the team is in the process of adjusting patient's pain and nausea medication. Today I consulted with the SW and she indicated that she will explore the possibility of music therapy.

- This chaplain offered deep listening, support, and reassurance to the patient, who expressed appreciation for the visit and requested me to return.

Suggested improvements

The patient, referred by SW, is a 50-year-old female end-stage cancer patient whose intense pain was compelling her to shift her body continually, unable to find a comfortable position as she awaits adjustments to her medications. The patient seemed to be feeling very low and was slow to engage in the visit but a deliberate conversational pace seemed to help build trust, enabling her to reflect on various aspects of her life. She emigrated from Kuwait when she was 17 and now is struggling with a sense of isolation, having only one close relative left, a brother, Samuel, who comes from there frequently on business. The chaplain offered patient gentle guidance and consulted with the SW who indicated that she will explore the possibility of music therapy. The patient expressed appreciation for the visit and requested a return visit.

- *Goal:* I plan to return tomorrow with a CD player for music and watch for an opportunity to address the patient directly about her hopes for living as well as possible until she dies.

RATIONALE FOR SUGGESTED IMPROVEMENTS
While story communicates more richly than phrases, brevity and simplicity are also primary considerations. Balancing the two is a frequent charting task.

Finding words

Perhaps the most frustrating aspect of writing chart notes is finally finding the descriptive words to convey spiritual care information. Some caregivers possess a natural aptitude for describing people and a well-developed vocabulary, but many do not. Most all of us who profess to become or remain spiritual clinicians need to continually work on diction, syntax, grammar, and especially creativity in use of imagination and intuition to describe patients and family members usefully. Focusing on the unique stories they tell will invariably provide the energy and enthusiasm for doing so.

Even fine writers struggle with their diction, as itinerant writer Jack Kerouac is reported to have said—one day he would find the right words and they would be very simple.

THE MERCIFUL ART OF SUMMARIZING
Nobody reads long chart notes. Oh, there are occasions in which several paragraphs are necessary for portraying the patient situation in unusual detail. But even those will not be read by more than a few IDT members directly involved and already appreciative of that unique patient situation. When professionals debrief colleagues about a given patient, only necessary details are included. There is a specific art of debriefing peers and supervisors that avoids burdensome extraneous detail and emphasizes the uniqueness of the situation. All professionals need to continually cultivate that art, especially leaving most self-reference behind.

People who have engaged themselves successfully in clinical pastoral education can suffer from another of its limitations in establishing a spiritual care practice. Writing down and processing disclosures about patients, in peer groups of that CPE learning crucible, teaches a budding chaplain to include his own feelings, attitudes, values, and assumptions in providing fullness of communication for the benefit of furthering self-awareness for their own personal and professional growth. But such self-centered detail does not fit at all in patient charts. It is actually annoying to busy, decisive, and dedicated professionals, who can quietly disdain them as burdensomely irrelevant red herrings. One such comment in a chart note can detract from the reputation of the writer and even from the professional image of the field of clinical ministry.

UNSHARED FEAR

Chart note

The patient is a pleasant woman in her mid-40s. She is lying in bed with her cell phone in her hand. Her room is virtually filled with flower arrangements. She welcomes the chaplain in, speaks readily and easily. Her faith tradition is listed as Jewish, but she indicates that she is "fine with interfaith chaplaincy." The patient reports that she was raised Jewish and her parents are, but that she is "not very spiritual." The patient tells the chaplain her medical narrative, she has been trying to cope with her diagnosis for six years and is increasingly frustrated and stressed by ongoing setbacks. The medical team is searching for new solutions. Patient: "I have lots of support, a great family and friends and my fiancé who is wonderful. But they are always saying how strong I am, how loved I am, and how I am going to be OK. I know they are trying to be supportive, but I am really scared. They don't want to hear how I really feel, they can't."

- The patient is facing a possible liver transplant and is frightened by the prospect of having to take meds for the remainder of her life. She has experienced loss of her independence, work life, and is also grieving the fact that doctors have told her she will never be able to give birth. The patient becomes tearful when talking about these losses.

· The patient speaks of how she is tired of feeling "lousy" all of the time. "It makes me mad and I have been feeling angry at my fiancé lately. If I have to stay sick like this, I am not sure I want to do this." The patient relates a story about a good friend who died recently of cancer at 50 years of age. She says, "She elected not to have treatment. I just know my family can't hear my feelings about that either."

· The patient is experiencing spiritual/emotional distress, she reports not feeling heard or understood by her loved ones, not affirmed in ways that would help those most important to her hear the emotions that are under her words. This impacts their effectiveness as a spiritual/emotional resource for her and likely negatively affects this patient's health holistically. The anger she feels is affecting her relationships. This writer did not explore with the patient, "I am not very spiritual." This is for ongoing pastoral care.

· Chaplain provided deep listening, affirmation, and acknowledgment of the patient's story and related feelings. The patient becomes tearful. Chaplain explores with the patient possible ways of building support as she moves forward in this situation— identifying a trusted listener who will sit with the patient's feelings, though they are painful. It remains to be determined who is best for this role of healing listener—a rabbi or a social worker, her fiancé or other person. Chaplain explores with the patient how it may feel to ask her fiancé and family members about their willingness to listen more, give advice less. Chaplain encourages the patient to continue asking for support. Chaplain writes referral for unit chaplain to follow up. Chaplain reads the patient's chart and notes that SW has already made a plan to see this patient and is aware that chaplaincy has been consulted.

Suggested improvements

This is a 40-something non-practicing Jewish woman who says she is "not very spiritual" and is beleaguered by six years of cancer treatment and numerous setbacks to any satisfying recovery: "If I have to stay sick like this, I am not sure I want to do this." She speaks easily of how fearful she is and how the relentless supportive comments from her fiancé and family members leave her misunderstood, alone, and internally angry. She grieves the likelihood that: she will never give birth, faces liver transplant surgery, and will have to take medication for the remainder of her life. The chaplain listened extensively and explored with the patient what it might be like to talk directly to her family and fiancé about her fears and her desire to talk openly with them. The chaplain offered to accompany the patient in a meeting with the family if the patient so desires.

- *Goal:* The chaplain agrees to inform other chaplains about the patient's need for ongoing support and possibly to explore with the patient her feelings regarding her religious and cultural heritage and the prospect of re-engaging them for her own benefit.

RATIONALE FOR SUGGESTED IMPROVEMENTS
Excessive verbiage burdens IDT members. This chaplain's intuition may have led her to engage the patient more courageously in offering further assistance with her family, fiancé, and religious resources.

FASHIONING RECOMMENDATIONS AND
PLANS (GOALS OF CARE)
Perhaps the most difficult among the tasks involved in spiritual care charting is that of making recommendations and formulating plans. Since most pastoral care in hospital settings is currently encompassed in only one visit with any given patient, any plan in many cases would

have to be carried out by somebody other than the assessing caregiver. Goals-of-care language is now to be used to fashion a plan of care. Chapter 3 includes many suggestions to consider when forming a spiritual care plan in bullet point form.

A plan is focused on what the *writing caregiver* is planning to do. It does not commit anybody else to action nor promise what somebody else will do. Recommendations, on the other hand, can be focused on what the writer thinks *others* could do to improve the specific patient's care. No generalized recommendations offered to improve the hospital unit functioning, to augment a hospital policy and procedure, or such global issues as enhancing medical education, improving nursing practice, enlightening theology schools, or upgrading government funding of caregiving programs are ever appropriate in the medical record. Find other places for your global opinions.

A FINAL EDIT: DELETING SELF-REFERENCE, THE TANGENTIAL, AND THE IRRELEVANT

A last cursory glance over your note before hitting "enter" should find any irrelevant stories, tangential comments and unnecessary self-references. Delete them. The time-worn advice to students of writing, "Strangle your darlings"[6] applies here. Take a brutal attitude to your well-written phrases that feel so good to write but don't really apply to the healthcare situation. That includes repetitive phrases that document your conversation with the patient, but convey nothing of use to any other caregiver in caring for that patient, including your spiritual care colleagues.

CPE experience for some spiritual caregivers left them with excessive focus on self-exploration—such things as what they were doing and thinking prior to an encounter, why they were late in arriving, how they ordinarily function with patients with a given diagnosis, or details about what they observed as they entered the patient's room. Such

---

6   Commonly attributed to William Faulkner as part of his teaching of writing students, and conveyed to me by high school English teacher and librarian Sister Mary Beatrice RSM.

comments were useful during training when the focus was on their own inner processes for learning about themselves as caregivers. But most self-reference is loud noise in the medical record. The focus there is on the patient not the caregiver.

Some patient stories are interesting and colorful, but have little or no relevance to that patient's human spirit regarding the current hospital situation. The term "relevant" derives from the Latin *relevans* meaning "to lighten" or to "relieve." Whatever doesn't cast new light onto the problem at hand or relieve tension about it in some way is not likely to be useful. Tangential comments "lightly connected" to some aspect of the situation are likewise more annoying than useful.

Well-known writer James A. Michener, author of such massive novel tomes as *Alaska, Centennial, The Source* and *Tales of the South Pacific*, is said to have once quipped that he wasn't a very good writer but an excellent rewriter. Taking half a minute to look carefully at your chart note before leaving it more often than expected will show changes you would like to make.

A final aspect of the charting process involves recording *outcomes* of the caregiving conversation. Outcomes are becoming increasingly of interest to regulators, insurance companies, and government funding agencies. Spiritual caregivers are to some degree participating in that movement, to evaluate patient outcomes and thereby devise interventions that seem by research to work best. Charting notes may become central to that branch of research, for the evaluation of individual chaplains, chaplaincy departments, and eventually the clinical ministry field itself. A phenomenological approach to recording and studying patient outcomes is presented in the next chapter.

6

Outcomes

A Phenomenological Approach

However beautiful the strategy, you should occasionally look at the results.

AUTHOR UNKNOWN (OFTEN MISATTRIBUTED TO WINSTON CHURCHILL)

As cartoon characters Frank and Ernest are finishing a round of golf, one refers to their scorecards and says to the other, "I never realized what a bad golfer I was until somebody else kept score." That quip fits chaplains of the latter part of the 20th century. Until then, because of the assumed confidentiality of their work, nobody seemed to think of evaluating the intricate aspects of what happened between them and the patients they served, and the results of their patient conversations in particular. Then a collision occurred in society between efficiency, accountability, and research fervor on the one hand, and the rise of interest in generalized spirituality on the other. Efforts mounted to find clarity about what chaplains do during their workday and to study its value. During the next decade scores of research studies pursued a way to prove that spiritual care adds actual value to the patient care and missions of healthcare systems (Flanelly *et al.* 2011).

While that evolutionary thrust of researching the effects of spiritual care continues, another effort to gauge effectiveness based on the nature of spiritual care makes sense as well. That is a phenomenological perspective that emphasizes direct observation of a patient's visage and tone before and after caring conversations. *One bullet point in chart notes can be used as a comment on what the caregiver noticed about the observable effect of the conversation on the patient.*

Defining outcomes of care for common spiritual needs (what pleases chaplains and what saddens them)

Such an approach starts with creating a model of outcomes that experienced chaplains like to see after addressing particular identified needs. The tables below show outcomes originally generated from focus groups of chaplains in the spiritual care department of a medium sized West Coast healthcare system. They were told that their project was to create a list of desired outcomes for each of the 21 spiritual needs[1] that were then being used to organize their charting. They were asked two questions to guide their discussions:

1. What specific outcomes do you hope will be observed in a patient after a conversation in which this need is addressed that makes you feel a little better when walking away after it?

2. What saddens you when you do not see it? In other words, what are some outcomes that you hope for that make you a bit disappointed when you don't see them?

The results of this rather extensive process are summarized in the tables below, corresponding to the four axes of spiritual needs

---

[1]   Several of these outcomes have been augmented considerably by the author after some years of experience using them. At the time that project used a list of 21 not 22.

described in Chapter 3: emotional support needs; major loss needs; religious and spiritual practice needs; and referral needs. The needs themselves are described briefly in the figures, on two levels. The first is intended for patient information material, aimed at an estimated level of understanding by 11-year-old children. The second is directed at an estimated level of understanding by healthcare professionals.

Note that the tables include a column entitled, "outcomes for research." This title refers to the potential value of conducting careful research in the future about the outcomes and their relationship to patient satisfaction, length of stay, and possibly cost savings of including spiritual care into treatment regimens on every service. To do that research would require accepting the subjectivity of spiritual care observations and their personal integrity in reporting them. To the degree that one would acknowledge the reality of such subjective bias, the research would add some convincing data to the purview of managers and administrators who are seeking to document the human benefits of identifying and meeting spiritual needs of patients and families.

These outcomes were designed to facilitate chaplains' evaluations of their patient visits. However, the identified outcomes also served well to promote chaplain and student awareness of what they were doing as they conversed with people exhibiting the various needs. Understanding the preferred outcomes reportedly made them more conscious of the process of their visits and tended to add substance, strategizing and depth to their patient conversations.

Axis 1: Emotional support need outcomes

1. TRAUMA SHOCK: PERSONAL SUPPORT FOR STABILIZING WHEN
FAMILIAR PATTERNS ARE DISRUPTED BY A CRISIS EVENT

Spiritual need	Outcomes for research
Patient view: You may need some help to put your day back together and find the next things to do when some very bad surprise has happened like your car accident or shocking news about somebody's health.	A patient or family member: • observably increases relaxation, e.g. facial muscles, eye contact, voice tone • engages in conversation for initial verbal processing of the event • expresses immediate emotions and/needs • participates realistically in immediate planning • contacts a support person for him/herself or has one contacted of her/his choice • accepts/requests prayer with chaplain or other spiritual leader • thanks the chaplain for stabilizing assistance.
Professional view: A spiritual caregiver sometimes has a role in trauma care, largely with family and friends, especially those who are present in support of the traumatized patient. The need often extends however, to the patient herself, including providing current orienting information, receiving and facilitating emotional expression, responding to religious perspectives, and contact with support persons. A calming presence, even with little effective activity, makes a contribution to trauma care when decision making is necessary about what to do next.	
After the trauma care, hearing the story of the traumatic events and its enduring results in the victim's life, from the victim's point of view, helps integrate the trauma into the life of the victim. The need for "debriefing" of staff members falls largely to spiritual caregivers, social workers, and specially trained group debriefing individuals if they are available.	

2. NEED TO TALK/EXPRESS: NEED TO BRING CONCERNS INTO VERBAL PROCESSING (INCREASE EMOTIONAL CONNECTION)

Spiritual need	Outcomes for research
Patient: It often helps just to talk and express yourself when things aren't going well. Chaplains know how to be with you, listen to what you are going through, and help you get more connected with people who care about you. *Professional:* A non-anxious personal presence that creates an interpersonal context in which patients can talk from their own point of view and get better connected with the circle of people who know and love them is the hallmark of chaplaincy.	• Rapport established, as patient begins to talk openly about herself and her situation in story mode. • Patient expresses at least one emotion clearly, whether named or not. • Patient becomes cognizant of the chaplain as a human being, making a personal comment about her. • Patient mentions at least one person—family member or friend—who cares about her in her current situation. • Patient expresses gratitude.

3. FEAR OR ANXIETY: NEED FOR REDUCING EXPECTATION OF IMMINENT OR PERVASIVE HARM (INCREASING HOPE)

Spiritual need	Outcomes for research
Patient: It is scary to have a condition that is serious enough to have to enter a hospital. Other things may make you fearful too, such as how this will affect you from now on or how it affects other people and things like your parents, your children, your pet(s), or your job. *Professional:* Fears range all the way from apprehension to paranoia, anxiety from feeling nervous to the persistent discomfort of a mental health disorder. A caregiver with a persistently calm, non-anxious presence is a start to reducing fear and anxiety, and in acuity can facilitate a possible referral for medication assessment.	• A calmer face. • Slower or more fluid movements. • A growing receptiveness to information and supportive, physical touch. • Acknowledgement of positive transcendence, such as a request for, or receptiveness to, prayer. • Connection to a loved one. • If severe, acceptance of professional assessment for anxiety medication or counseling. • Expressed gratitude.

Spiritual need	Outcomes for research
Patient: When something bad happens to you your natural reaction may be to be angry, at many things, some that don't even seem to make sense. A chance to tell somebody freely just how bad your situation is and how you feel about it, may help. *Professional:* Anger is a natural part of loss, the incursion of medical need, and even prolonged or acute discomfort. A person who listens patiently with eye contact, understands (at least partially), receives the anger, sorts its origin to the degree possible, and responds realistically may reduce the level of aggression. Security and law enforcement officials may need to be present or near.	Observing *the angry person:* • Hearing the person's verbal expression of anger and his best understanding of the reason(s) for it. • Restraint from acting out or escalating. • Eventual receptiveness to the limitations of life inherent in the people, situations, or events at which the person, present or past, is angry. • Improved perspective on the complexities of the angering situation or events. • Gratitude expressed.

5. SADNESS, DISCOURAGEMENT, DESPAIR: NEED TO RAISE MOOD AND/OR INTEGRATE LIMITATIONS

Spiritual need	Outcomes for research
Patient: Everyone has bad days sometimes but some things make us much sadder than that, and can even make us feel like not going on with our lives. It can be hard to get courage and a smile back into us with any liveliness at all. *Professional:* Assessing a patient's level of discouragement, all the way from mere sadness at disappointing events to suicidal thinking is a necessary function for quality care when marked sadness is observed in a patient. Either encouraging with positive yet realistic interaction on the one hand, or promoting referral for mental health assessment on the other remains the decision and its follow-through options.	• Patient appears seriously sad. • Patient acknowledges the sadness. • Patient shows awareness of the reason(s) for the sadness by beginning to disclose one of them. • Patient responds to conversational assistance to expand on the specifics of the reason(s) for the sadness. • Patient acknowledges the realistic scope of the sadness as painful but not overwhelming. • Patient mentions another person who might understand the sadness. • Patient accepts referral for professional assessment of depression if indicated.

6. PERSONAL HURT: NEED FOR UNDERSTANDING OF PERCEIVED PERSONAL MISTREATMENT

Spiritual need	Outcomes for research
Patient: Big changes and bad treatment by people hurts deep inside. You may feel it in your heart or your stomach. That hurt can last for a long time and won't be understood by very many people. It is very, very difficult to talk about. Please try though, because that is how it starts to get better. *Professional*: Hurt generally hides under anger and fear. Feeling slighted by a caregiver feels re-wounding in the midst of the high vulnerability of hospitalization. Some levels of hurt can be assuaged simply by sharing. To salve a patient for hurtful interactions she received while in the hospital, providing a realistic perspective on the natural limitations of health care may help at this level. At the other end of the spectrum, however, rape, combat, abuse, and child neglect change the core of people and their stories get collapsed into a few words, never to be spoken. Such traumatic events may need very specialized treatment, but may spurt out raw in the context of a caregiving relationship. They first need a hearing, and then maybe referral.	• Patient responds at least cautiously to queries about what lies beneath her fear, sadness, or anger. • Patient acknowledges the hurt. • Patient tells a story about an event that hurt her. • Patient expands on the story or tells others. • Patient converses about hurt, anger, and/or fear as related and troubling (conceptualizes). • Patient responds to queries about previous help received for the situations and events that hurt. • Patient accepts professional assessment for having experienced abuse or neglect. • Patient expresses gratitude for the conversation.

7. EMPOWERMENT: NEED FOR HELP TO IDENTIFY AND USE ONE'S OWN NORMAL OR IMPROVED PATTERNS OF COPING

Spiritual need	Outcomes for research
Patient: Sometimes you need help to find your own best self in a tough situation. *Professional:* At times people regress in the face of difficult situations, i.e. they seem to take refuge in an earlier stage of development, losing their best coping selves momentarily. Regression can be the chronic pattern of a dependent personality or the normal shock of crisis or trauma.	A patient: • in a real or perceived crisis allows and receives the presence of a calm caregiver • discusses his/her coping, including the way(s) s/he has previously coped with difficult situations • indicates increased realistic insight into her condition • mentions or explores options • expresses or shows increased awareness of the limitations of healthcare systems • expresses appreciation for presence and quiet understanding.

Axis 2: Major loss care outcomes

8. GRIEF SUPPORT: RECENT OR IMMINENT MAJOR LOSS

Spiritual need	Outcomes for research
Patient: Finding out that somebody or something important to you is suddenly gone or soon will be makes people feel mixed up with being mad, sad, scared and loving all at the same time. That is called "grieving" and chaplains know how to help with it. *Professional*: Major loss presents a classic spiritual care project of assisting a person facing the situation of recently or immanently having something treasured taken away, probably forever. Currently grieving persons employ a wide variety of coping methods. Discerning them taking place and facilitating them as best we can helps the beginning of integrating the loss into his/her life.	Receives assistance with one of the named coping mechanisms, i.e.: • visible emotional expression (e.g. sad faces, angry tones, tears) • quiet shared reminiscing • religious practice or ritual • communal supportiveness • love expression • realistic decision-making or planning • efforts at reconciliation.

9. GRIEF COUNSELING: RECURRENT DISTURBING EMOTIONS FROM PAST LOSSES

Spiritual need	Outcomes for research
Patient: Saying goodbye can take a long time. A hospital can give you memories and remind you that you may not have said goodbye enough for something that happened long ago. Chaplains know this and they know how to help you continue saying goodbye. *Professional:* Chaplains recognize quiet grieving of past losses and respond with a careful listening ear and gentle questions that promote the reminiscing that can further integrate the loss into that person's life.	• Mentions previous loss. • Expresses emotion. • Receives validation. • Shares reminiscences. • Cries while talking about the lost loved one. • Considers referral for further grief assistance. • Expresses greater hope.

Spiritual need	Outcomes for research
Patient: When doctors, nurses, and the whole hospital can't help you anymore, you may be dying. When you realize that you are near the end of your life you may need help with how to finish things in your last weeks and days. You many want help to say goodbye to everyone and everything you love.	Openly discusses an "end of life" issue such as: • afterlife • relationship with the Divine • pain control • reconciliation with estranged loved ones • life review • forgiveness of sins/regrets • religious membership/practice • concern for survivors • bereavement of other family members • organ donation • discussing burial arrangements.
Professional: Palliative care and hospice care prepare people for a good death and can be highly complex. Many people do not have such preparative attention, however. When there is no time or availability for such care people can still be helped with the dying process as soon as it includes a new realization that it is now happening. Discerning what an individual's unique needs are for life resolution and doing what one can to assist him/her with the projects that prepare them to die well remains a fundamental spiritual care project.	

11. ADJUSTMENT COUNSEL: MAKING PEACE WITH A MAJOR CHANGE IN FUNCTION OR APPEARANCE

Spiritual need	Outcomes for research
Patient: Very bad things that happen to your body often change your life forever and you'll have to get used to the situation. Chaplains can help you get ready for living the new ways you will need for the new way things will be. *Professional:* Chaplains partner with people who need to adjust to recent or past irreversible negative changes in function or appearance, by listening, empathizing, understanding, and sometimes suggesting, to help the integration of the new levels of functioning into the person's life situation and personality.	· Mentions need to adjust. · Verbalizes or shows feelings about the life-changing situation. · Discusses or openly considers some of the implications of the change. · Considers options for adjustment. · Demonstrates a more positive perspective, verbally or nonverbally.

12. RECONCILING ESTRANGEMENT: HOPING FOR AND RESISTING RETURN TO POSITIVE EMOTIONAL CONNECTION WITH SOMEBODY YOU LOVE

Spiritual need	Outcomes for research
Patient: Hospital care might remind you that somebody has been hurt or mad at you for a long time and that you really want to see them again. Chaplains can help you do what you can to heal the distance that keeps you apart. *Professional:* Illness or injury often brings back to consideration open personal conflicts that have distanced and even estranged people from one another. Need occurs when patients and family members seek to reunite with specific people who have either felt or caused personal hurts in the past. The chaplain serves as a transitional facilitator of reconnection, and when possible, healing of previously strained or estranged relationships.	• Mentions an estranged relationship. • Talks openly about the estranged relationship, particularly "what happened" to estrange them from one another. • Agrees to receiving contact with an estranged person of importance to him/her. • Agrees to initiating contact with an estranged person of importance to him/her. • Acknowledges having "done enough" to seek reconciliation, even though it is felt unlikely to be accomplished.

Axis 3: Religious/spiritual practice needs outcomes

13. RELIGIOUS SUPPORT: NEED TO FEEL THE POSITIVE PRESENCE OF TRANSCENDENCE

Spiritual need	Outcomes for research
Patient: When you are really scared, sad, upset or confused, you might want somebody to pray with you or talk with you about God. A staff member, chaplain, or other spiritual leader can help you feel like you are surrounded by God. *Professional:* The world's great religions have developed spiritual practices that have lived for centuries for their ability to help some people feel the positive presence of transcendence in difficult life circumstances. Providing religious support through prayer, ritual, sacrament, and liaison with the patient's valued spiritual leader usually helps to fill this need, at least temporarily.	The patient: • prays with the chaplain or support person • receives a sacrament • receives a spiritual ritual • is contacted by a spiritual leader of his/her choice.

14. SPIRITUAL VALIDATION: NEED TO SHARE UNIQUE WAYS ONE NURTURES ONE'S HUMAN SPIRIT

Spiritual need	Outcomes for research
Patient: There are many different ways of being spiritual and not all of them fit with the ways churches usually believe. When you are in the hospital you may want to share with somebody those things that really make your mouth smile and your eyes shine. *Professional:* A variety of spiritual practices and convictions that support the lives of people are not closely related to traditional religions. Persons with significant non-traditional spirituality elements may need to verbalize with excitement practices and beliefs they highly value. Someone who hears their value to the patient and validates that value cares spiritually for that person.	• Talks with animation about a spiritual self-care belief, practice, or experience. • Receives conveyed empathy validation of the efficacy of the practice for that person. • Acknowledges or facially appears validated and understood through calming.

15. SPIRITUAL COUNSELING: WONDERING ABOUT CHURCH AND TRANSCENDENCE

Spiritual need	Outcomes for research
Patient: Things that shake your heart can make you think new thoughts about God and church and make you wonder about God and what you learned before. Talking about your questions or bad memories of religion with somebody who won't make you feel like you should do something their way can help you get peaceful again.	• Openly discusses spiritual questions or problems, such as religious practice, a spiritually supportive modality, religious/spiritual concepts (e.g. heaven, hell, God, salvation, forgiveness, sin).
Professional: When people are physically compromised they may need to discuss religious matters, questions, problems, issues, and past harmful events.	• Mentions, shows emotion about, or begins to process disenchantment with a religious organization.
	• Asks deepening questions of apparent core life concern.
Most of us carry with us a history of religious learning, practice, convictions, and disenchantment with religious organizations and leaders, some of which can impede using religious and spiritual support for healing. A positive experience of a religious representative that is supportive, reconciling, and healing may help clarify the very sensitive issues that have grown around religious teaching and experience.	• Shows tears or otherwise expresses emotion of awe, anger, hurt, regret, resentment, or peaceful joy.
	• Expresses interest in continuing to explore in some way the issues raised.

16. LIFE REGRETS: NEED FOR RELIEF FROM GUILT OR SHAME

Spiritual need	Outcomes for research
Patient: When serious things happen, thinking about your past decisions can cause you to regret parts of your life that you wish had been different. Usually what we wish we hadn't done or said cannot be changed or improved and needs to be shared in order for us to feel better. Even when the persons we hurt can't forgive us, we can learn to mostly let go of the bad feelings inside ourselves. *Professional:* Guilt is a perennial spiritual issue, a natural prodding from within that we have caused harm to another or humanity itself. Shame is feeling bad about ourselves as inferior or deeply flawed, especially in a way that others can see. Care for guilt and shame can be intricate, but it involves offering a process to move towards accepting what one cannot change, softening the self-punishment of guilt and shame from past actions or neglects.	• Mentions or shows need for forgiveness in dialogue. • Confesses regrets/"sins" with some degree of openness. • Receives words and/or signs of reconciliation. • Refers to God or Allah, or hears forgiving words from a caregiver. • Appears observably more relaxed, positive, or hopeful.

Spiritual need	Outcomes for research

Patient: When you are worried or scared, some basic ways of calming and getting OK with the situation can help, like praying, and understanding things better.
 	
Professional: There are a variety of self-care modalities that can be taught briefly to help meet the emotional upset of a difficult life situation. Expertise in providing these varies considerably among even certified spiritual caregivers.
	• Receives instruction in one of the following:
	
	  – advanced directives
	  – medical ethics
	  – chemical dependence
	  – sacraments
	  – devotions
	  – the rosary
	  – meditation
	  – guided imagery
	  – healing touch
	  – relaxation exercises.
	• Smiles or observably relaxes.
	• Verbally reports improved understanding and/or acceptance.
	• Expresses gratitude.

Axis 4: Referral needs outcomes

18. ETHICS CONSULTATION: NEED TO UNDERSTAND OR DISCUSS TREATMENT OUTCOME CONCERNS

Spiritual need	Outcomes for research

Patient: Sometimes the doctors and nurses need to talk with a family to help them make a big decision about your health. You might want somebody to talk with you about your own understanding about it.	• A person:
	  – expresses confusion or dismay at the apparent medical options
	  – openly discusses an ethics question or perceived dilemma
	  – participates with family member(s) in an ethics consultation
	  – communicates having clearly made a medical ethics decision.

Professional: Ethicists have developed principles that help people decide along with healthcare professionals what is the best way to proceed with very difficult medical conditions. At these joint decision times spiritual caregivers might bring unique perspectives to the meeting, such as knowledge of underlying family dynamics, their previous history of dealing with right and wrong decisions, a family member's deep personal convictions, specific religious teachings, and regrets/resentments left over from prior painful life decisions. Teamwork in combining empathy with realistic perspectives to find and communicate the best options remains a palliative care art.	• Patient/family members demonstrate, verbally and attitudinally, resignation to the limitations of health care and the human body.

19. ADDICTION OR MENTAL HEALTH CONCERNS: HAVING INNER WORRIES ABOUT YOUR DRINKING, DRUG USE, OR BEHAVIOR, OR THAT OF A FAMILY MEMBER

Spiritual need	Outcomes for research
Patient: Being hospitalized can be a chance to get help finding the right counselors when you have secret concerns about your own drinking, drug use, sad feelings, or odd behavior. You can also get to share about your family's drinking or bad actions to help you understand it and maybe help them.	• Participates in a calm conversation about the person's emergent problems.
	• Sharing on any level of the patient's own concerns about mental health symptoms or the patient's concerns about the consequences of his/her addictive behavior.
Professional: People suffering with addictions and/or mental illnesses, whether previously diagnosed or not, can benefit from a non-moralizing, caring focus on the specifics of their own concerns about the consequences of their behavior. Facilitating such referrals can be very difficult but life-saving, since very few IDT members will have the skills and interest in dealing closely with very troubling people. Skills needed are careful listening with specialized frameworks of understanding that keep the emphasis on the patient's own concerns, focused querying, and networking with professionals of other disciplines.	• Sharing of chemical use or behavioral concerns about a family member.
	• Acceptance of assessment by a qualified addictions counselor or mental health professional.

Spiritual need	Outcomes for research
Patient: Everybody sometimes has serious concerns about their romantic partner and these can be made worse by being in the hospital. Just talking to somebody confidential about it can make you feel better. *Professional:* This need is for understanding, advice, or referral about hurtful problems affecting one's love life. A person's primary relationship affects and is affected by everything else of significance that happens to him. As a major aspect of the spirituality of most people, intimate relationships can bring considerable personal pain. At those times we can benefit from sharing and getting consultation, which may lead to receptiveness to further professional care. Hospitalization presents an opportunity to do that.	• Expresses negative feelings about one's lover's wellbeing or the relationship itself. • Speaks openly about the relationship and situation. • Considers referral for counseling assistance.

21. ADVOCACY: NEED FOR SUPPORT IN FINDING ADDITIONAL NEEDED CARE

Spiritual need	Outcomes for research
Patient: Sometimes people who could help you don't know you need the help or are so busy they don't know what you need. You may need somebody with you to figure out what you do need and help you find it. *Professional:* Some patients are quietly disappointed with the care they are receiving, feeling neglected by the healthcare system or specific caregivers and unable to speak about it. Regardless of the quality of care they receive, some patients and families need assistance to verbalize and sort out their concerns. Dependent personalities chronically feel neglected and harbor unrealistic expectations of help that is available. The need may be to listen and facilitate patients and caregivers to move towards mutual understanding of what is in the best interest of patients and within the limitations of systems of care. This can be very difficult work.	• Concerns about care expressed. • Increased appreciation for the limitations of health care. • Alternative care identified and received. • Staff apology received if indicated. • Increased satisfaction expressed. • Increased self-responsibility acknowledged.

22. FAMILY CONFLICT FACILITATION: FEELING CONFUSION OR ANGER AMONG YOUR FAMILY

Spiritual need	Outcomes for research
Patient: When you're sick sometimes family members disagree and argue. You may wish you had somebody to listen to them, make suggestions, help them talk together, or call a family conference to figure out the situation. *Professional:* The seriousness of healthcare situations can cause family conflict or rekindle previous conflicting family issues. Care is then for a caregiver to absorb anger and facilitate communication in families who currently disagree or are confronting longstanding resentments among them. If listening is impossible, or the issues are too complex, the situation indicates working towards referral to another, better-prepared professional.	• Family conflict expressed, even subtly. • Conflict noted verbally by a family member or caregiver. • At least one component of the conflict explored openly in conversation. • One family member shows new understanding or willingness to address conflict. • Accepts assessment for counseling. • One family issue reaches some measure of resolution.

Qualitative studies: Assessing outcomes

While no quality research has been done using these concepts and processes, a few quality improvement studies were completed regarding what percentages of which outcomes were seen in conversations about 8 of the 21 needs. The studies for crisis care and end-of-life care are shown in Tables 6.1 and 6.2 as examples. In those studies chaplains were asked to complete a data collection sheet after each time they addressed specific identified needs to be studied. The data sheets listed the hoped-for outcomes and chaplains simply checked whether they saw or heard that outcome in the conversation. The tables illustrate the results.

For example, the need called "crisis ministry" (now called "trauma shock") was studied for two weeks as chaplains used the data sheet to record observed outcomes. They were asked to not merely record their impression of the outcomes impulsively, but to ask themselves if their impression of what happened in the conversation would have been seen and heard by anybody standing beside them for the entire visit. The following percentages were found in the obviously small quality improvement study.

Table 6.1 Outcomes of crisis care events

Observed outcome (N=44)	n	%
Emotional needs expressed	40	91%
Conversational engagement	40	91%
Support person contacted	34	77%
Realistic planning	25	57%
Increased relaxation	36	82%
Prayer requested or accepted	31	70%
Expressed gratefulness	21	48%

Note that the titles of the needs studied differ from those in Chapter 3. That is because the list of outcomes has evolved through experience over time to better reflect the development of thinking about outcomes. The results suggest that most of the time the people in these crises were able to talk with a spiritual caregiver and expressed emotion in doing so. They seemed to relax somewhat in conversing, at the 80 percent level. Over two thirds of them contacted a familiar support person and engaged in prayer, showing that their cognitive functioning had become at least minimally active. Over half were able to actually plan for what would come next and were interpersonally sensitive enough to thank the caregiver.

A second need studied was named "End of life care" at the time, which in Chapter 3 is called simply "Dying." In the early 2000s palliative care spread rapidly through US hospitals, vastly improving the dying experience of suffering people in hospital settings. Many people still die in hospitals, however, without hospice and palliative care or before it can be initiated. The following study was a two-week effort by hospital chaplains to look closely at the outcomes of their conversations with people approaching death in a general hospital.

Table 6.2 End-of-life care outcomes

Observed outcome (N=32)	n	%
Openly discusses an "end of life" issue such as:		
Bereavement of other family members	23	72%
Love expressed	22	69%
Religious heritage/practice	21	66%
Afterlife or relationship with the Divine	19	59%
Life review	18	56%
Concern for survivors	16	50%
Reconciliation with estranged person	14	44%
Burial arrangements	13	41%
Organ donation	7	22%

Note that the patient mentioned concern about the grief of other people and expressed love of somebody during the visit about 70 percent of the time. Religion and the afterlife were part of the discussion in about two-thirds of the conversations. Estrangement was mentioned a surprising 44 percent of the time. These data, even with such a tiny population of cases, prompted some suggestions for the spiritual care team's continuing education and team discussions about improving care.

The major obstacle to confidence in this method of evaluation is quite clearly the universal human penchant for self-deception. The difficulty of being reasonably objective in catching the subtle signs of either satisfaction or disdain in the subject of one's own spiritual care is at least some level of a barrier to using this method. However, clinical pastoral education, the formative program of professional chaplains, has been furthering development of optimum objectivity in chaplains' observations through peer group feedback now for almost a century.[2] Fully certified chaplains can reasonably be assumed to be at least a bit more objective making observations about personal and interpersonal matters than the average person. And while this method of evaluation remains highly subjective, it should be acknowledged that objectivity is always only (to a point) in any clinical discipline, and indeed even in quality research projects.

Preparation for spiritual caregiving as a professional has long included efforts at developing a mind with enough fluidity of focus to move quickly from conversation to appraisal of how the interaction went. Called "self-supervision," that capacity involves the intricate practice of taking a final few seconds of most patient visits for reflection on the outcome, asking oneself what happened to (or inside) the

---

2   Professionally facilitated peer supervision that optimizes clinical students' direct validation and critique of their actual patient conversations remains the hallmark of ACPE accredited CPE residency programs that are still the primary formational education of certified professional chaplains. Regular feedback fostered in CPE has the intended effect of a participant growing in awareness of how others see him and his ministry work as juxtaposed to how he has been seeing himself. A degree of objectivity gradually shaves off habits of hyperbole, minimizing, and other forms of distortion in how one observes oneself in relationship. There are obvious limitations and wide diversity in the ways in which students make use of that crucible of self-exploration and especially in how they become convinced of the value of continuing that practice after training.

patient during it. Making observations of what may have changed in a patient during a depth of care encounter is a valuable component to communicating about that patient in writing.

Obviously authenticity and rigorous integrity are crucial here, to reduce excessively sanguine rosiness, minimizing denial, and "awfulizing" about negative conversational patient responses or otherwise distorting what one has seen and heard. It is easy to assume somebody feels positive about you simply because he showed no animosity to you. It can also be easy to feel judgmental about oneself or a patient at slight impressions of rejection. The compliance often shown by vulnerable people may not go very deep, belying the authenticity somewhere beneath. Social level compliance easily hides underlying feelings, issues, and needs.

In addition, self-deception of caregivers themselves always remains an aspect of our humanness, no matter how much we invest in consultation and clinical supervision. Virtue has been mostly neglected in assessments of applicants for certification as chaplains and in the peer reviews of chaplains, even chaplain supervisors (Hilsman 2010). As ethicists are discovering though, without virtue there is not much value in standards, research, and demonstrated knowledge (Pellegrino 1993; Pellegrino and Thomasma 1993).

A caregiver's honest intention and robust efforts to record only what he has observed that would have been noticed by anyone else standing by may be the best we can do to keep phenomenological evaluation of outcomes reasonably realistic and accurate in chart notes. Occasionally making patient visits in tandem with a peer or supervisor, followed by open mutual feedback, does help. Making such duos gender mixed may limit buddy collusion but certainly won't eliminate it. Like any observational process this one too can be developed and continually learned. Regular consultation helps immensely to retain adequate objectivity in a necessarily highly subjective practice (see the Epilogue).

The subjectivity here parallels the visual assessment that accompanies almost every medical encounter and nursing diagnosis in daily appraisal of the patient's personal health condition by simply looking closely at her. It also is congruent with the cursory, variously conscious look we humans make in our every encounter with a friend, a spouse, and our children. In that quick grasp we are intuiting the mood, attitude, and emotional temperature of that person with whom our relationship is significant to us. With intentionality and practice we may even be catching any differences, if any, in our impressions before and after the conversation. Nobel Prize-winning psychologist Daniel Kahneman has written insightfully about when to trust the intuition of a highly experienced professional. What he calls the "two systems," loosely equivalent to what have been called intuition and cognition, work together in a quick process to enable us to know something without knowing how we know it. While these quick impressions of patients are often of little value to patient care, sometimes they are substantive and occasionally they are strikingly relevant to a patient's condition and life healing.[3]

The simple studies illustrated here could be expanded into quality research projects. The benefits of that research would be to further develop understanding of the processes involved in addressing each of the needs and the importance to patients and the system of meeting those needs. It would ground the learning process of students and chaplains as a method of improving their awareness of the dynamics involved in a focus on spiritual needs in patient visits.

Studying outcomes in these qualitative ways has at least two advantages. It helps motivate caregivers through the human interest generated. And in continually developing these outcomes we are moving to the point at which quality research will render agreed-upon convictions about best practices and evidence-based spiritual care, however temporary those may be.

Quantitative studies: Analyzing incidence and its implications

Focusing on described spiritual needs can also be useful in research using a more quantitative approach. We can use numeric data to

---

3   "Expert Intuition: When Can We Trust It?" in Kahneman (2011).

study the incidence of the various needs identified in a given hospital unit, individual chaplain's practice, and healthcare system as a whole. Almost no research has been conducted on using the set of concepts presented in this book in this way. But efforts at quality improvement have been initiated, and we hope to show here that quality research would be possible and beneficial to the field of clinical ministry.

Electronic medical records (EMRs) can be altered to organize data—about how many patients admitted into a given hospital service were recorded to have been seen as fearful, for example, or grieving past losses, or markedly angry about some aspect of their lives, including the life position in which their medical condition has placed them. EMRs can crunch data as to which chaplains identify specific needs such as addiction concerns, ethics confusion, or family conflict more or less often than their colleagues, and eventually relative to benchmark standards. Quality improvement studies based on this data, designed specifically for a given healthcare system, become sources of information that guide manager decisions about chaplain deployment, administrator goals in oversight of various departments, and chaplain team collaborative engagement about how to address the spiritual needs of each patient care unit.

A few healthcare systems have already begun to do this with their chaplain staff. They set up the EMR software in a way that can provide useful data on what specific kinds of care would not be provided if a given hospital unit were to reduce the staff by even one chaplain, for example. They have also used data summaries to determine which chaplains may need continuing education for a better understanding of, and improved skill for, addressing any given need.[4] This simple quality improvement process has documented the needs for spiritual care in various hospital services of one hospital system during a period of over ten years. Figures 6.1–6.4 illustrate some of that value for spiritual care managers, quality officers, and administrators.

---

4   See the Epilogue for how personal issues of caregivers can partially blind them to seeing, and therefore identifying and recording specific needs.

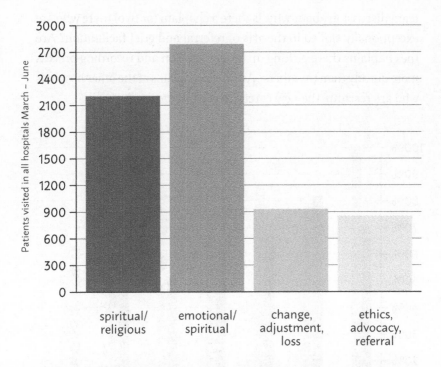

Figure 6.1 Incidence of the four axes of spiritual needs recorded system wide in March 2016

Figure 6.1 illustrates the results of a pilot quality improvement study of the incidence of the four axes of needs over some months in early 2016. A total of 894 patient visits warranted chart notes through the medium-sized health system that averages 5700 discharges per month. Figure 6.2 illustrates the percentage of patients visited that received interventions for needs observed in the four axes, organized by system facility. The chaplain turnover in that system was unusually high because of recent retirees and rehires, as well as the ordinary turnover of CPE residents and interns. As they were learning the recording system, the EMR showed data that compared each hospital to the other five in how many patients received interventions for each category of need. Note the high numbers of referral needs and loss needs at Hospital 3, which is the smallest of the six hospitals. That revelation could catalyze team discussion about why. Is there a chaplain (or two) there who are exceptionally skilled in the arts of referral and grief facilitation? Are the chaplains there picking up the recognition and recording process more quickly than the others? Are there chaplains at the other hospitals who are resisting the new careful recording system?

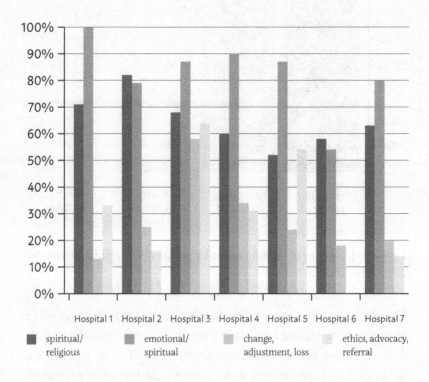

Figure 6.2 Incidence of spiritual needs by axis and system hospital

Figure 6.3 shows a comparison of intervention types for the four spiritual needs axes organized by level of chaplaincy experience: staff chaplains, most of whom are certified; CPE residents who are in the midst of a year-long formative clinical education process; and CPE interns who are functioning as student chaplains in a beginning clinical learning experience. When adjusted for the time each type worked in direct patient care, this study would serve as one measure for productivity, one criterion for deciding on what mixture of chaplains and CPE students may be best. It tests the assumption by hypothesis that experienced chaplains recognize specific needs more effectively than students, and residents better than interns. When studied over time, the hypothesis that CPE students improve in their recognition of the various needs over the course of their involvement in the CPE program could be tested as well.

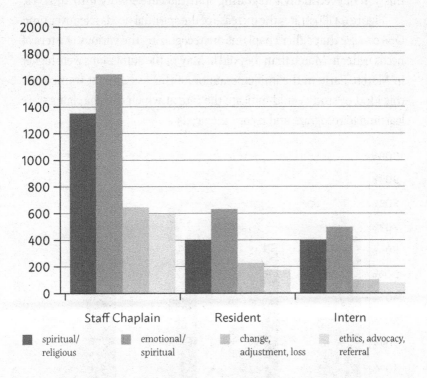

Figure 6.3 Chaplains, residents, interns

Note that in general the expected data configuration occurred. Staff chaplains recorded more interventions than residents, who recorded more than the interns in every category of need. More detail is needed for this data to be meaningful, however. How much time did chaplains in each category work? Presumably the staff chaplains dedicate more of their time to patient care than residents and interns, who have heavy educational involvement along with their patient care. Also knowing which staff chaplains are full time and have extensive other duties to perform would further define the comparison of these three levels of spiritual caregiver. The management at that facility has cogently resisted tying chaplain performance to time spent, however. If lingering remains a key factor in patient disclosure then incentivizing *more* patient visits in a day rather than *quality* ones would be counterproductive to the mission of eventually integrating spiritual care solidly into all IDTs.

Figure 6.4 illustrates the increase of the spiritual needs axes over time. One can see that either chaplains are recognizing the various clusters of needs better in March than they did in May, or the admissions were higher in March. Early in the implementation of this assessment framework, this kind of study could indicate the rate at which the chaplains were learning to recognize and record the needs.

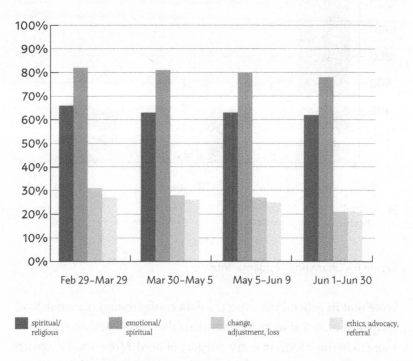

Figure 6.4 Rate of learning or change over time

Clearly all of this relies on trusting that the chaplain staff do not, consciously or unconsciously, "pad" the notes to improve their being seen in a more positive light by spiritual care managers and mission leaders. Isn't that true of a fair amount of spiritual care research in one way or another? At the very least, studies that employ chaplains' recording of their perceived outcomes of their own patient conversations offer a manager data with which to help shape staff meeting agendas and annual chaplain evaluations.

This hospital system's spiritual care leaders later chose to record interventions rather than needs. Interventions are then assumed to be based on patient needs. But documenting needs keeps the focus more obviously on patients rather than spiritual caregivers. Managers, administrators, and particularly governing boards and the public would seem to be more deeply interested in the spiritual needs of their patients, especially those that go unmet, than on what their chaplains are doing.

Quality control and quality improvement studies are still more influential locally than hardcore research. Professional quality studies can seem to board members to be remote and different from the local facilities, not directly representative of the local scene. On the other hand, local quality improvement studies that look at hard numbers of patients in that geographical region who exhibit specific painful life situations can tweak a humanitarian bone in conscientious leaders.

Style differences among chaplains show themselves boldly in some such studies. Two certified chaplains, both women, of similar age, long-time friends, working in hospitals of similar size in the same healthcare system, experienced that boldly. Their profiles of what needs they documented over several months differed significantly on one need—love-life pain. One documented that need extensively and the other not at all. That revelation challenged the one to look more closely at why that would be so, improving the comprehensiveness of her charting of spiritual needs, as well as at her own attitude about a love life being seen as spiritual.

Besides the drawback of the self-deception of chaplains rating their own patient conversation outcomes, there are other weaknesses to this phenomenological approach. So far no way of tying observed outcomes to material factors (costs of care, money saved, etc.) has been devised. Not everything valuable has a positive monetary result. There is, as yet, no verifiable research proof that identifying spiritual needs improves medical or nursing care. Those still remain in the anecdotal research area, where stories of patients who have benefited from recognizing needs and addressing them abound and could be gathered into essays.

In the entire process of writing useful chart notes and evaluating their outcomes one is wise to guard against becoming too algebraic. Ambiguity characterizes all spiritual care. Expecting too much precision, comprehensiveness and certainty in any comments on the human spirit can quickly become distracting, tedious, and unrealistic. Spiritual care is an art, like the practice of medicine, not to be burdened by excessive expectations of vigorously scientific proof regarding what is essentially an endless mystery.

Epilogue
Becoming and Remaining a Spiritual Clinician

A spiritual clinician is *a person who uses direct observation, interpersonal encounter, and developed frameworks of understanding to augment the human spirit and clarify the religious complexities of people in difficult life situations.* There are both skills and personal characteristics that allow a person to succeed at that work. Some of them have been standards for decades in the primary chaplain certifying bodies of the US, and some of them go beyond that traditional list. What follows is an educated guess at what is needed now and what is likely to be required in the near future.

A special set of skills for spiritual clinicians

Skills remain the basis for most success anywhere, necessarily augmenting luck, aptitude, nepotism, and gratuitous inheritance. Strategy, teamwork, leadership, and organized collaboration do contribute heavily to the success of sports teams and symphony orchestras, but nobody excels in those endeavors without well-developed basic skills. Similarly, no matter what certification one achieves, basic caregiving skills moving towards excellent ones are what give a caregiver the best chance of great success as a spiritual clinician.

The experience of chaplain associations in certifying palliative care and hospice chaplains during the second decade of the 2000s disclosed a few skills that many certified chaplains seem to lack, making them of little use in the integrated teams serving suffering and dying people. Here are essential skills for aspiring spiritual clinicians of any discipline today.

LINGERING

It is easily taken for granted that a caregiver can wait for the few seconds it takes to nonverbally invite a person to deepen her disclosure. A core aspect of listening—lingering— moves quietly beyond the social convention of responding quickly with your own point of view, or related experience, or supportive comment, or a clarifying question, not to mention a change of subject to something more interesting or comfortable to the listener. It implies interest in the speaker beyond what he is saying at the present moment. It allows just a bit of time for the other person's reflection that might deepen the next response. Experienced chaplains generally know but continually relearn its value in practice. Lingering is silence as a verb. It is interpersonal waiting. It is a strategically placed skill and a demonstration of genuine care at the same time. Filling the silence too soon truncates the possible emergence of deeper disclosure.

GRIEVING

Substantial skill at grieving, towards healing of one's own major losses, has recently been seen as a prerequisite for working in a palliative care or hospice setting. In those services, patients are losing so much that a caregiver who has not dealt effectively with her own life losses may well be missing a great portion of the grieving necessary to care for others. Ungrieved losses and complicated grief do not show themselves easily to those who have them, even professional caregivers. But there are indications of grief-need to sharp observers. And these can be used in certification processes (see the "Essential processes" sections below) to help them be found. "Can this person talk in a rather full manner about how he has dealt with the death of his father?" for example. Or, "What did he do with the feelings of grieving?" Or "Who knows of the depth of your emotions about that loss?" Helping an aspiring caregiver recognize the poorly grieved losses of his past and accept remedial help with the grieving stands as a pivotal gift.

NEAR UNIVERSAL RAPPORT (HUMAN-TO-HUMAN RELATING)

Establishing rapport is essentially relating to a person human to human rather than authority to subject. It is doing what one can to deepen an intersubjective relationship to allow a patient's disclosures about what is most important for her to say right now, beyond social interaction or compliance to professional practice etiquette. It requires personal characteristics such as a kind of confident earthiness, as well as skills including supportive comments, empathy conveyance, useful personal questions, and reasonably objective interpretations. In this context it suggests an ability to open up a relationship that produces intimate details in vulnerable sharing.

Medical and nursing clinicians' rapport is generally only what is enough to provide diagnosis and treatment recommendations. It can be rather narrow, involving only the purview of medical practice, not the broad range of both ordinary and crisis life struggles that constitute spiritual care. Both currently certified chaplains and practicing clinicians may need significant internal change to learn to relate human to human to almost everyone as spiritual caregivers. Without rapport there is little of value for a spiritual caregiver to write in the medical record.

RELIGIOUS UNDERSTANDING

One difficult cluster of competencies with its own knowledge base is religious understanding. To negotiate that complexity will almost surely require academic education into the history of world religions

SPIRITUAL CARE IN COMMON TERMS

with a concentration on one of them in some depth. Competency with a few functions of spiritual care can be acquired with a minimum of time, as palliative care physicians and nurses have found. But for other functions, especially caring for such religious needs as providing experiences of positive transcendence and sorting through the intricacies of religious abuse, church regulation resentments, and interest in remedial learning of church teachings, further clinical and academic preparation will be necessary.

PRESCRIPTIVE AND AUTHENTIC SHARED PRAYING

The skill of praying with people can slide into patterned pedantic subtle preaching. To be able to pray authentically and not merely sound serious it is worth guarding against the relentless human tendency for image management and over-control. Close, communal examination of written verbatim reports can sometimes reveal that student chaplain prayers are more like taking refuge in a comfortable action for the caregiver than meeting the patient in her current difficult uniqueness. Not everyone wants prayer, or needs it. Penicillin is a fine medication but passing it out to everyone in the hospital unit is surely not prescriptive. Regularly asking oneself a few hard questions tends to keep what seems like prayer, actual prayer. "Is this a real prayer or a dutiful effort to find fitting words?" "Did you take three seconds of self-reflection to bring this prayer out from your own soul?" "Is this indeed my prayer or just a nice prayer?" The ability to access one's own depths and address the profundity of a personal transcendence seems quite often to elude religious leaders either pervasively or unpredictably. In healthcare settings that authenticity becomes even more crucial to people facing the ragged limitations of life.

There are of course many ways of praying, ranging from a staid reading of prayers from books and reciting them as memorized on one end, to singing them and passionately proclaiming them on the other, with calm and thoughtful utterances focused directly on a patient's felt needs in the middle. The flexibility to use any of these authentically at any given time based on the guessed preferences of a given patient is a plus for professional spiritual caregiving.

There is also the art of making shared prayer prescriptive. Does this prayer fit this person right now? Does it penetrate to the core of the current concerns of this person as you have come to understand her? Indeed, does this person even want to pray with you now, despite her polite acquiescence to your invitation to pray? Sorting out what the interest in, habits of, and need for shared addressing of a person's image of a positive transcendence takes a bit of quick intuition and experience. But as the premier spiritual action of most human beings, prayer that fits them can fill a huge hole in their day and make an unforgettable contribution to a healing process.

CONVEYING EMPATHY

A staple of chaplaincy over the decades, showing a person that you "get" what they are saying on an emotional level, almost defines spiritual care (see Chapter 3). It is not likely to have been a focus in either medical or nursing education, however. And while some individuals convey empathy rather naturally, most of us do not. No matter how much we feel for another person, getting that reality across to them remains more difficult given our communication patterns developed in and since childhood. It may take significant practice to develop this skill, replacing diagnostic listening with personal listening which seeks access to the soul.

MASTERY OF ASSESSMENT FRAMEWORKS

Spiritual clinicians possess ways they have consciously established to ground their care. All spiritual caregivers are using conceptual frameworks in their appraisal of patients. How else do they know what to say next? The question is, how aware are they of the frameworks they are using? Simplistic religious frameworks such as being saved or not, being right with God, and having a personal relationship with a savior, are clearly not adequate once a caregiver enters the complexity of actual patient issues. Becoming clear on at least some of the concepts and convictions that guide your caregiving is part of the skill base of a spiritual clinician. There are innumerable frameworks for assessment that have been developed by hospital chaplain teams during the early 2000s. Adapting one or more of these for authentic use in assessment, or fashioning a viable one of your own, is a choice of developing spiritual clinicians. To do this established chaplains have examined, at least to some degree, their unconscious ways of measuring people and developed new ones more functional in recognizing spiritual needs.

ASSESSMENT

Literally meaning "to sit with" (Latin *ad* meaning "right up next to" and *sedere* meaning "to sit"), the term implies that one needs to sit with a person for a while before making any substantive reflections on his spirit. The word "assess" is used here primarily because it is less definite than "diagnose," yet refers to getting a picture of a person's human spirit and its needs when compromised. Being able to appraise a person's spirit in a way that is both tentative and useful to other caregivers is foundational to spiritual care in a clinical facility. Why else make a spiritual assessment than to help the other caregivers working there understand and respond to the current needs of that person's heart? The mysterious nature of the human spirit is such that appraising it is always very partial, temporary, and tentative. But it can be very useful to maintain the humanity of patients and, for some caregivers, to guide personal and interpersonal care.

DOCUMENTING

This entire book is directly about this function, documenting the care provided. As a verb, from the same Latin root as "doctor," "to document" means to teach by actual written evidence. As a noun it refers to an official written instrument, example, proof, or lesson—or chart note. In a given note the key questions are what are you trying to teach by this document and to whom? Writing clear and relevant medical record chart notes is one of those essential skills. The art of describing people and their core concerns succinctly in the immediate context of their medical predicaments is indispensable for any clinician wanting to expand her care of the spiritual aspect of people. Such description is the key skill that can be learned, a project for which this entire book has been dedicated.

Writing succinctly and accurately about people is one indispensable skill of this emerging profession of clinical spirituality, and the longstanding discipline of clinical chaplaincy. Adequate writing suffices, as long as it communicates sufficiently well to IDTs. Excellent writing of chart notes is a goal to pursue for all of us.

FLUIDITY OF MOVEMENT FROM THE CONCRETE TO THE METAPHORICAL AND THE CONCEPTUAL

Learning conceptual terms for complex phenomena such as grieving, celebrating, reminiscing, and the various levels of denial, allows for efficient communication. Recognition of metaphors a patient uses unconsciously to convey what her situation is like allows a depth of understanding that left brain analysis never knows. Some competence in these two directions uses intuition and adds to it in empathically connecting with a patient on the emotional level. A measure of mastery of the use of concepts and metaphors, along with the ability to linger, brings a depth of earthy maturity to a caregiver. Lack of these abilities leaves one's care rather one-dimensional, sometimes one-issue, and tending towards formulaic. Beginning CPE students are urged to become aware of their repetitive phrases in caring conversations so as to increase their ability to allow disclosure to take its own course towards deeper trust. Useful summarizing in chart note writing emerges from such fluidity of sensate, cognitive, and intuitive perspectives.

Personal characteristics (essential virtues)

A spiritual clinician's identity includes, beyond skills, a number of personal characteristics not common to whatever previous positions she has held. Human development is enormously complex, and nobody is born a spiritual caregiver. So everyone purporting to be trusted as one will need to change significantly inside, to let formational processes affect her deeply, allowing the making of a new identity. She will need not only to learn things but let herself be changed by the personal and professional formation the new role requires. Skills and communication techniques boldly fail when personal characteristics limp. As medical ethicists learned long ago, the clearest principles, best-defined policies and most comprehensive protocols lie useless when virtue has not found its way into the core of a practitioner. Personal characteristics are what constitute practitioners' perspicacity, their unique perspectives from which to view complex situations. Here are a few characteristics that are indispensable in budding spiritual clinicians.

SPIRITUAL MATURITY
One needs a bit of spiritual maturity in order to deal helpfully with the spiritual issues of another person. Given our pragmatic definition of spirituality, spiritual maturity can be defined as *habitually living with generalized acceptance and frequent joyfulness on the edge between the strictures of excessive certainty on the one hand and the overwhelming alarm and anxiety of tragedy on the other, as one daily faces an uncontrollable world.* In other words, spiritual maturity is the capacity to stand in the ambiguity of life while continuing to function with confidence and consistency.

AN OBJECTIVE EYE
Physicians, nurses, and social workers all base their professions on direct observation and other focused and defined data—from radiological imaging, lab tests, text book diagnostic frameworks, journal-published research studies, family member descriptions, and verbal patient histories—to prescribe or plan for what is best for this person in this situation. Spiritual clinicians seriously consider data from interpersonal encounter over their own deeply held beliefs and established theological convictions, to guide patient care in meeting the limitations of human living. That includes looking at each patient

The quality of having a ready insight into things; clear-sightedness; shrewdness as a unique and elegant human being worthy of caring rapport and objective description of personality, life situation, and current needs.

A SPIRITUAL CARE IDENTITY

Throughout this book we have implied that specific members of professional disciplines other than trained chaplains can serve as spiritual caregivers, even clinicians who are simultaneously functioning as physicians, nurses, and social workers. That assumes the development of a spiritual care identity. How a clinician will become competent as a spiritual caregiver today seems only to be done well in the small group, self-explorative, supervised program of experiential program called clinical pastoral education. The characteristics and skills described below are worth considering in any map of progressing through such a program, as well as the lists of competencies in current use by chaplain certifying bodies.

We need a brand new identity for spiritual caregiving, and nobody is born with it. It is generally developed through an intangible process during a period of patient care under close examination by peers and an experienced educator. Long known as a pastoral identity, it can be defined as *a solid sense of oneself that lends confidence and consistency in providing spiritual assessment and care to any person in spiritual pain.* Of course confidence without competence is dangerous to people receiving care. Certification processes work to evaluate competence in people who are already confident that they have it.

A COMPETENT, CONFIDENT COLLABORATIVE SPIRIT

The ability to work together with other professionals as colleagues, neither expecting too much of them nor of yourself, can be a characteristic that is difficult to acquire. It may take years to do so. The desire to collaborate well is a prerequisite. Collaboration requires knowledge, congeniality, tolerance, easy forgiveness, assertiveness and spontaneous communication clarity. It supplants tendencies to work in relative isolation with either a mild victim or superior aloofness.

RADICAL SELF-AWARENESS

The emotional availability that characterizes spiritual caregiving is based in large part on the emotional awareness of the practitioner. One tends to do to others' feelings what one does with one's own. If a chaplain tends to submerge his anger he'll likely be superficial with the anger of a patient. If she minimizes her fear in denial, her ability to be non-anxiously present to and supportive of a fearful patient is in question. Self-awareness has long been a staple requirement for certification as a chaplain, and a primary goal of CPE programs. But the level of self-awareness it has taken to be certified by chaplaincy associations may not be adequate for serving in some healthcare services today. The courage of repeatedly risking what it takes to become radically self-aware makes it easy to avoid, to stay elusive under normal emotional blindness, to which very blindness zealous aspiring spiritual caregivers can remain blind. This is a criterion for spiritual caregiving that must not be lost, and needs to be continually resurrected as a goal of would-be spiritual caregivers due to the ease with which it becomes lost by intellectualizing, self-deception, and absorption by organizational and political activity.

Self-awareness proceeds on two different planes: immediate awareness of one's own emotions in the moment, and ongoing familiarity with one's own life story as it has shaped one's relationships. The true meaning of the virtue of humility consists of neither seeing oneself as superior to any others on the one hand, nor being intimidated into inferiority to any one of them on the other. That describes a continually growing self-awareness that is always at risk of eroding momentarily through life's honors and challenges.

Engaging the stories of patients generally doesn't plunge very deep when a caregiver has only dipped his toe into the waters of his own life history. That is a phenomenon that cannot be seen until one has recognized the power of his own key life events in sharing them in some fullness with others. Talking openly about oneself is a prerequisite to actually hearing the complexity and sensitivity of others' personal stories. Those two movements occur intertwined in peer supervision and the dynamics of other sustained small group experiences. Other contexts for such sharing, normally found in romance, counseling, and some friendships, generally need to be enhanced by peer group experience focused on self- disclosure and interpersonal engagement.

A patient's attitudes, values, and life assumptions remain mostly hidden to caregivers who have not been shaken by stark revelations about their own. Just as the earthy nurse sees more in a patient's eyes and nuanced words than most neophyte RNs, so does any caregiver better grasp the relevance of a patient's inner responses to his predicament if she has visited the haunted rooms of her own hurts, disappointments, and failures. Experience in exploring one's own relationship history bestows on us a surprising capacity to catch the relevance of patient stories during this hospitalization and its healing/maturing potential. Literally meaning "working together," the word "collaboration" requires communication with and a flow of functioning together with other disciplines. Holding oneself above or below them in value is the antithesis of humility, which knows oneself and values oneself accurately, neither exaggerating one's specialness nor minimizing one's usefulness.

EMOTIONAL MATURITY

Awareness of your own emotions, enough to be fairly conversant about them at least when asked to reflect on them, is only a prerequisite to the maturity of employing one's feeling-life fairly consistently in caring for one's own relationships, both personal and professional. A close look at the relationships of all human beings would reveal holes left in our ability to use all of our emotions richly in our relationships. Some of us come out of our families unable to be angry, or show our hurt, or own our fears, or indulge our sadness. What we do to our own actual beneath-the-surface emotions we tend to do with those specific emotions of other people. If we habitually mute our anger, we'll not see much half-hidden rage in patients. If we typically hide our fears with jocular light-heartedness, we'll mostly miss the underlying fears of patients. Such deficits in our relating to people on a feeling level tend to truncate our functioning as budding spiritual clinicians. A fair amount of learning and training helps fill these partial voids in our emotional relating. Only honest interpersonal feedback, well timed and well worded, can show us these voids as motivation to fill them.

A useful piece of pragmatic spiritual psychology is that each of the primary feelings has a path from infantile primitive rawness towards mature use for enhancing life enjoyment and relationships. In the adult human they each span a continuum, based on what has happened to that human since infancy. Briefly, this highly complex reality can be illustrated by the continua below:

- *Anger.* "Anger management" programs help people of all social strata find ways of expressing themselves when highly aggravated or enraged, that are not likely to be destructive to people and one's relationships. Assertiveness programs, on the other hand, help people express themselves in ways that reach people with the offense or disgust that those people typically keep suppressed. Maturity with anger is relatively consistently being able to use anger as fuel to communicate what one doesn't like forcefully enough to be taken seriously, and not outrageously enough to be taken as pathology. A great deal of anger gets expressed in a healthy IDT and an unknown portion of it is transformed into resentment and hostility. Any spiritual caregiver needs maturity of her own anger to be able to work in that setting as a facilitator, receptor, container, and interpreter, without becoming either jaded or devastated. Nobody does any of this perfectly every time.

- *Sadness:* Maturity with the feeling of sadness hangs in the mid-range between the despair of total defeat on one end, and hard-hearted intransigence to people's misfortune on the other. Maudlin tones indicate the edges of the former and curt responses to sad events, the latter. Acknowledging sadness when it sweeps through you, without descending into the persistent discouragement of depression, shows the development here. Attending to actual depression as it encroaches by seeking help for oneself remains an element of the same maturity.

- *Joy:* Gushy melodrama and giggly histrionics, just short of clinical mania, truncate depth of relationships. They do connect with others in the same strata of affect prevailing at the moment. But until they run their course they preclude serious consideration of the situation at hand. On the other hand, humor and light-hearted rejoinders ease tensions and can allow fresh perspectives that are missed by burdensome over-seriousness. The skill of knowing when and how to celebrate and amplify the positive while tuning in quickly to the serious implications involved in the situation signals maturity in the emotion of joy. It is joy that makes life worthwhile, of course, as broadly speaking the only source of enjoyment there is.

- *Hurt:* Deep hurt is disabling, temporarily or sometimes forever, or until significant healing occurs. But for most of us most of the time, the project is how to meet the mid-level hurts that sting, discourage, aggravate, and spark retaliation. What is maturity in dealing with the normal slights and insults that result from an imperfect humanity? Making them too big makes you obnoxious. Making them too small by constantly ignoring them eats away at your self-treasuring. How to find the words to communicate about hurt feelings without having to display all of them all the time is the project of searching for maturity regarding this emotion. It remains the most neglected emotion in our everyday lives.

- *Fear:* Fear is there to warn us of danger, the encroachment of pain, injury, diminishment, and personal sabotage. Listening to your fear rather than denying it, and finding courage when you actually need it is a sign of budding maturity with fears. Ignoring your natural fears is no better than exaggerating them.

When meeting that armed gang member in the ER, your fear is instructing you to pay attention to that shiver rising around your ears and across your shoulders. And recognizing the anxious restlessness that surges quietly within you whenever a physician appears in your presence may be the best clue you have to discuss your attitudes about authority somewhere with a wise person you trust. Significant fear can be a striking clue to the way towards personal growth as you overcome the disabling fears and move on to more comprehensive ability to achieve rapport with almost any human being you meet. Fear can be seen as a clearer sensation than anxiety, and a frequent component of it.

- *Guilt/shame:* Guilt signals that you have violated some significant standard of behavior or even thinking that has been established inside yourself. You have hurt someone, or everyone. Remorse, the frozen stuck-ness of negative rumination, wastes energy that could be productive in the natural human pursuit of actual helping of other people and peaceful joy for yourself. On the other hand, guilt tells you something about your own imperfect decisions. Time and ordinary defences tend to mercifully cover our guilt about foolish mistakes and important neglects, but only a level of sociopathy sees no regrets at all in a personal past. To exaggerate your shame or guilt, as feigned humility that is actually negative pride, becomes quickly burdensome for anybody around. Using your guilt to inform you, acknowledging your failures when it fits a situation, and moving on to the more personal immediate context is maturity regarding guilt. The Tenth Step of AA states, "Continued to take moral inventory and when we were wrong promptly admitted it," to guard against the self-pity that may be just below the surface of preoccupation with regret and the self-doubt of shame and remorse.

RELIGIOUS CONFIDENCE

Religious convictions and practice still occupy a large segment of spiritual care work. When there is considerable upheaval in the religious life of a caregiver there are liable to be troubling lacunae in her ability to remain objective and useful in discussing serious religious questions with patients. This distortion is of course not absolute or certain. But some resolution of the universal questions that arise relative to a caregiver's religious heritage and subsequent personal pondering is necessary to quiet a mind when discussing the religious questions, however different, of another person. "What is prayer?" for example, and "What happens after death?" and "What is this transcendence we all feel and how does it regard me, if at all?" Such questions lie at the heart of some of the rumination common to hospitalized people. Having faced them oneself makes possible the assisting of verbalizing the "take" on them of somebody hospitalized.

Chaplains commonly remain peripheral to their religious organizations while maintaining deep convictions about the aspects of religion that do ground them. They remain open to virtually all ways of being guided through the currents of religious belief, ritual, and practice while rather vigorously maintaining their own. This could be termed religious serenity, except that one can also practice religious care at those times in life when serenity stands distant, elusive, and waiting for a change to make room for it to reappear.

INTERPERSONAL COURAGE

Lots of things go wrong in health care. But people continue to seek help with medical problems and probably always will. "The show must go on" quip from entertainment applies here too. Everyone eventually meets the limits of human care and dies. Healthcare facilities are full of tragedy. Some new scenario erupts unexpectedly and things go bad. These settings are not for the completely tender-hearted. There must be resolute sturdiness. There must be willingness to go into brand new territory at any given moment. There must be resilience, dogged persistence, suspending personal need and returning again and again to the fray. This stalwart virtue, classically called fortitude, is indispensable for all clinicians including spiritual ones.

DEDICATION TO THE PEOPLE AND THE WORK OF THIS TEAM
A fine spiritual clinician cannot remain aloof or peripheral to a treatment unit. While spiritual caregivers have no physical treatment role, no essential function to improve a deteriorating medical condition, they dedicate themselves to the spirit of the team as a whole and lend support—listening, debriefing, providing grief assistance and prayer in any immediate need situation, at any hour. They stand with the members suffering, even secretly, from their perceived failures, their mistakes, and their unrelated regrets of life. They recognize and honor the limitations of human care, the ideals of young caregivers, and move when possible to help people to acceptance of those limits. The word "dedicate," rooted in the Latin *de* meaning "away" and *dicare*, meaning "to proclaim, affirm, set apart" suggests here that one devotes time, energy, work, and passion for what is happening in this unit. This is more than just a job.

COMPREHENDING AND COMMITTING
TO CLINICAL SPIRITUAL CARE
Wanting to do good, help people, and contribute to the world is essential but not sufficient for functioning as a spiritual clinician in a healthcare setting. Neither are having a job, getting paid, maintaining a position of relative importance motivation enough. The clinical ministry movement is *a loosely associated throng of people dedicated to caring for the human spirit through direct relationship in a practice that is grounded in the behavioral sciences, spiritual conviction, and altruistic practice.* A score of professional associations support the movement worldwide towards an eventual goal of relative equality of healthcare focus on body, mind, and spirit. Why would an aspiring spiritual clinician not commit to that movement, rather than only to her own life satisfaction through competence and good work? Commitment

to that movement is especially important by anyone serving as a leader in the associations that support it. Short of that there is only commitment to his own professional associations, denomination, or self-aggrandizement.

Essential processes: Gaining competence

Certifying bodies variously recognize that quality spiritual care evolves with society. For example, while there are basic and advanced skills that are likely to remain fundamental forever, such as personal listening and conveying empathy, new skills are needed now for integration of spiritual perspectives into the daily work of specialty IDTs. As society continues to develop, our understanding of people, communities, relationships, and medical issues must also evolve. The pertinent question is, "What are the skills and characteristics needed for this age to work with satisfaction and effectiveness in hospital IDTs?" What follows below is an experienced, intuitive guess in answer to that question.

In order to develop the identity and skills of a spiritual clinician, people engage several interpersonal processes that further the development of their practices and their careers. The accepted ways of acquiring these have been those developed by the clinical pastoral education programs in medical, mental health, parish, corrections and addiction facilities, mostly across the US. Most of these modalities of learning and development still stand as essential today. Here are brief descriptions of some of the traditional ones that could well be augmented for the evolving field of clinical ministry and a few new ones that are becoming necessary.

CLINICAL SUPERVISION

A useful definition of clinical supervision is: *the careful exploration of actual spiritual care relationships in a context of trust and respect, with a knowledgeable and experienced mentor, for the purpose of establishing caregiver identity and gaining further competence.*[1] Similar to psychotherapy, it differs in focus. Therapy aims at improving one's relationships and living quality through healing, while supervision centers on the subject's caregiving relationships of assisting the healing of others.

Clinical supervision in this context is organized as a small group experiential process whose chief objective is to process verbatim reports of the group members' spiritual care conversations. To do that in a consistent way that is as objective as possible, it uses three distinct kinds of group sessions: verbatim sessions, didactic instruction sessions, and interpersonal relations sessions to facilitate, manage, and learn from the peer relationships that develop in the group. Traditionally it includes group facilitated evaluation sessions aimed at clarifying group members' learning issues and descriptive final evaluation documents that help them focus learning goals for the next phase of their education or work life.

SMALL GROUP IMMERSION

CPE is always conducted at least partially in a small group format. Supervisors facilitate group interaction for the personal growth processes and care competence of students who have contracted for the educational value of programs. "Small group" generally means four, five or six students, since above that size programs begin to lose the small group dynamics that optimize peer feedback, a primary objective of CPE programs. The facilitated small group dynamics phenomenon that almost forces qualified people to become honest with one another about their self-images has been the genius of CPE programs' success at preparing people for spiritual care work.

---

1   The ACPE, the generally recognized premier association of clinical pastoral education supervisors in the US, and the only one authorized by the US Department of Education, defines its mission as "A community of professionals committed to nurturing connections to the sacred through experiential, transformational education and spiritual care."

PEER SUPERVISION

In the small group interaction of CPE groups, each member is a peer colleague expected both to *offer feedback* to other members and find her own vulnerability in *receiving feedback* on her own spiritual care relationships (Tartaglia 2015). So far no other field has maximized peer supervision as significantly in its formational education.

A THEORETICAL BASIS

Some scheduled educational time in CPE group education is dedicated to didactic instruction, to continue a process of establishing frameworks of understanding people and the various ways of offering help to them. Developing one's own theory of spiritual care, not merely incorporating that of somebody else, is a major project of preparation for becoming a spiritual clinician. Many theories and helping modalities are presented to group members by various professional disciplines as pieces useful in fashioning their own. Some educational engagement with other disciplines remains a standard for CPE programs.

CONSULTATION

Literally "to strike together," the word refers to courageously opening up one's inner processes to trusted colleagues in order to gain insight and possibly new direction of one's care of a given person. Learning to consult is the primary learning goal of CPE group interaction. Its regular practice is also the primary function for maintaining one's competence as a spiritual clinician over the decades of a career.

Essential processes: Demonstrating competence

How is a manager or administrator to know which of 26 applicants for a spiritual care job to hire? What are the lenses through which she can peer to reduce that pool to three who she will interview? One of those is the certification history of the applicants. Which ones have been certified and by which chaplaincy associations? Before meeting the applicants, a manager has the option of knowing that certified people have faced a small group of their experienced peers expecting them to show that they have largely mastered skills and developed characteristics that optimize the likelihood that they can succeed in a spiritual care role worthy of being paid for it.

The primary associations of chaplains in the US[2] have been evolving standards of practice and identifying essential competencies as qualifications for certified members for at least 50 years (Hemenway 1996).[3] Their processes for assessing whether or not a person has mastered these criteria continue to churn as well, with the assumed purpose of minimizing caregivers' own issues—pretension, self-deception and the little excessive self-indulgences that tend to sabotage genuine care and rigorous self-reflection in practitioners.

Now it is becoming clearer that some other competencies need to be emphasized for chaplains to fit integrally into IDTs and make substantive contributions to their work, along with continuing their individual care of pained people. Some improvements could be made to that process, and we offer some suggestions here. But essentially that way of confirming the readiness of a person to start functioning professionally as a chaplain will and should remain the basis for any evolutionary improvements ahead. What needs to change? Two things: first, certification would be better accomplished in an interdisciplinary context. This has been tried in some certification processes for palliative care chaplain specialists. That model could be expanded. Chaplaincy needs greater integration with other clinical disciplines, and including informed members of those disciplines in certification interviews would be a real, albeit small, movement in that direction. A certification team of some combination of perhaps two chaplains, two nurses, a physician, and a social worker would have promise of gradually eradicating the somewhat insular nature of spiritual care

---

2   The Association of Professional Chaplains (APC), Neshama: Association of Jewish Chaplains (NAJC), and the National Association of Catholic Chaplains (NACC). The Canadian Association for Spiritual Care (CASC) parallels these together in Canada.

3   The ACPE was formed by the incorporation of four already functioning regional associations in 1967.

in hospitals that pervades at the present time. Logistics and possible payment of some certifiers could be arranged by leaders who are convinced of the great value of that change.

A second suggested improvement would be in the number of competencies an applicant is required to address in that brief certification hour, which itself could well be longer.

A two-tier set of competencies could be sufficient to approve adequacy of practice of an applicant. Some currently required competencies could be approved by paper submission of the applicant writing to show understanding of a competency and examples of how she has demonstrated it in her work. Examples of these are medical ethics understanding and involvement, documentation in the medical record, and conceptual understandings of group and organizational behavior.

Other competencies, however, need appraisal face to face in real time with experienced peers. The capacity for comprehensive human-to-human rapport needs to be seen during the certification hour. Pursuing the grief history of the applicant, the practice of spiritual assessment, excellent self-awareness, emotional maturity, and how she incorporates her own attitudes, values, and assumptions into her caregiving work are examples of such competencies that ought not to be certified without vigorous face-to-face engagement.

The value of interpersonal engagement as a staple of certification processes remains great, a breakthrough in quality assurance, and cannot be lost. But as in all professions, some people who have been certified are later shown by behavior to either have been mistakenly certified or else to have slipped beneath adequate quality of functioning into impairment. Maintaining competence as a spiritual clinician will always be an ongoing project given the natural deterioration of the human by age.

Essential processes: Maintaining competence

Two singular processes need attention by those certified individuals seeking to maintain their authorization to function by spiritual care associations, even as those associations themselves change their focus, shift their organizational relationships, evolve, and continue to reduce their jousting with one another.

First there is the need for spiritual caregivers to dedicate themselves to constant learning. This needs to be more than words and beyond mere compliance to regulation. Current chaplain associations maintain requirements for numbers of hours per year of continuing education, and some standards for what those hours entail. The responsibility for ongoing development of one's profession still lies solidly with individual practitioners, however. Certified spiritual caregivers need to be vigorous in developing their own plan for a number of years to further develop their competence in specific areas; address personal characteristics that are troubling; and otherwise address weaknesses in their practice. We all have them.

The second essential function for maintaining competence is partially communal. It is developing and maintaining vigilance for impairment in oneself and in one's colleagues. Certification only determines competence on a given day, often early in a practitioner's career. Impairment is a reality. It descends upon us like the proverbial thief in the night. Suddenly it is there. We only recognize it at the mention of a trusted friend or an uncommonly forthright colleague or official. It helps to realize that if we work long enough all of us will become impaired in one way or another.

Vigilance for impairment is only a third of the way to the uncommon care it takes to meet the need of a colleague who is becoming impaired. Another third is courage. One steps into a perilous place when one decides to bring forth to a peer observations of his possible burgeoning impairment. Only a few physicians ever do such intricate caring in their discipline. A doctor friend says that everywhere he has worked there are medical practitioners on the staff to whom other physicians would never refer their daughters, mothers of friends. Almost all colleagues simply don't think carefully about that possibility in their peers. And when they do recognize dysfunction, they fail to follow through for lack of courage. It is easier to simply let another's failure confirm one's own self-impression of superiority and go on one's way.

The final third of a quality impression of a colleague's impairment is skill to negotiate that first conversation. Once you see it and summon the courage, there is the chasm of words that won't come. Practicing the scene with a savvy other person, a counselor perhaps, or a seasoned colleague or chaplain, can serve as a temporary mentor.

Be prepared to fail at first. Hardly any of us would respond positively on first brush to anyone noting that we are becoming in even some small way incompetent. What works with people with drinking problems, the "intervention," is never done by one person alone. Done well it always works. Not that the subject always accepts assessment or treatment, but in some way it places the issue so directly in front of the eyes that it begins to ruin any pleasure or comfort the addiction still provides. We owe one another this greatest moment of care.

And let us generate the persistent humility that will allow us to hear when that time comes to face our own overarching limitations.

Conclusion

Some 23 centuries after Hippocrates separated clinical medicine from belief modalities of helping, health care is quietly thirsting for a clinical discipline capable of looking at spiritual experience with a broad, knowledgeable, and objective eye, and communicating about it in common terms. Additional skills are needed now for the close collaboration of clinical disciplines in care of the human spirit that is emerging as a core need in healthcare culture. Palliative care, hospice, and addiction treatment are some of the specialty services that have found the need for practitioners capable of focusing on both religious and broadly conceived spiritual needs in conjunction with the other clinicians with whom they work. Patients in general hospitals can benefit from these additional spiritual care skills as well—from the focusing of interdisciplinary communication effectively on the spiritual aspect inherent in the human makeup.

Appendix

The Use of Chaplain Chart Notes by Interdisciplinary Team Members at a Leading US Hospital

Gordon J. Hilsman, D. Min. ACPE/NACC Supervisor with residents Samsiah Abdulmajid, M.A., Michael Bousquet, M.Div., Amanda March, M.Div., Barbara Schreur, M. Div. and Heather Lucas, M. Div.

Abstract: Reports on a quality improvement study of interdisciplinary healthcare team (IDT) members at a major US hospital regarding how often they read chaplain chart notes and access them for insight into the spiritual states of patients and families in their care. It also includes IDT members' assessments of three characteristics of the chart notes they see: whether the notes tend in general to be understandable, substantive, and useful. Data are arranged by professional role of respondents.

Introduction

The professional discipline of chaplaincy in a hospital optimally focuses on the character, state, and practice of how patients care for their own human spirits, as well as any current spiritual needs operative in them during the personally challenging experience of hospitalization. Chaplains are engaged in efforts to listen, gain rapport, convey empathy, identify needs, and address them, communicating the content and substance of these efforts in their clinical notes. To the degree that such communication doesn't happen, the spiritual aspect of patients' needs remain shrouded, and spiritual care, no matter how skillfully provided, is seen as an adjunct, peripheral intervention. Chaplains who consistently make meaningful contributions to patient care, and who chart these observations and interventions in terms easily comprehended by IDT staff members become integral members of the interdisciplinary care team. Thus this study begins inquiry into the effectiveness of chaplains' notes for IDT members by providing an anecdotal baseline for how comprehensively chaplain chart notes are read and accessed for insight by IDT members.

Electronic medical record (EMR) systems, in spite of their myriad problems, have significantly contributed to patient care by centralizing multidisciplinary patient information in one place, by eliminating difficulties with legibility, and by lessening the physical work of interacting with a patient's information. However, regarding spiritual caregiver notes, there remain major limitations within EMR systems. Limitations due to constraints within the EMR system (restrictive options of checking boxes and using phrases rather than sentences for example), and limitations caused by poor narrative charting skills (use of religious jargon, excessive self-reference, cryptic brevity, and unnecessary generalizations) continue to render some of the notes almost unusable by IDTs. To what degree can established chaplains be motivated to seek continued improvement in their charting skills? Will statistics about how much interest their notes generate in staff members raise that level of motivation?

Purpose

To study the use and usefulness of chaplain medical record charting notes to IDT members in selected hospital nursing units.

Study context

NCH (fictitious name) is a fully accredited 1000-bed facility, employing 4100 nurses and about 4000 physicians and residents. It regularly achieves designated status as a top research organization. Its care has long been considered to be world class, as confirmed by top ratings among all US hospitals. It admits 48,000 inpatients per year for an average overall length of stay of 5.8 days.

The hospital employs seven full-time interfaith chaplains of whom six are board certified. The work of the full-time chaplains is augmented by trained per-diem chaplains, volunteer ministers, and five chaplain residents enrolled in a year-long Association for Clinical Pastoral Education (CPE) accredited residency program. The six certified chaplains have served the hospital for an average of about 15 years and are well integrated into the fiber of their assigned units.

Methodology

This was an anecdotal baseline study, not intended as professional research. A survey instrument was designed specifically for this project by a CPE supervisor and six CPE group members. The residents and an intern personally presented the instrument to a self-selected variety of interdisciplinary care team personnel during day and evening shifts on hospital inpatient units. Some of the instruments were similarly presented at IDT staff meetings. Potential respondents were told that completing the survey was optional and that it would take about a minute to complete it. Residents received the completed surveys, which were then collated, tallied, and analyzed. The data were then arranged in tables shown below, sorted by hospital unit and healthcare provider role.

Results

Table A.I shows the respondents' estimated level at which they seek chaplain notes for insight into their patients. Table 2 shows respondents' estimates of how often they read chaplain notes when they see them.

Table A.1 IDT members who seek spiritual care chart notes

	n	Most of the time		Often		Hardly ever		Never	
RN	86	12	14.0%	32	37.2%	34	39.5%	8	9.3%
MD	12	0	0.0%	4	33.3%	7	58.3	1	8.3%
Other	18	2	11.1%	2	11.1%	10	55.6%	4	22.2%
T	116	14	12.0%	38	32.8%	51	44.0%	13	10.3%

Table A.2 IDT members who read spiritual care notes when they see one

	n	Most of the time		Often		Hardly ever		Never	
RN	86	27	31.4%	33	28.4%	20	23.3%	6	7.0%
MD	12	2	16.7%	5	41.7%	4	33.3%	1	8.3%
Other	18	2	11.0%	7	38.9%	5	27.8%	4	22.2%
T	116	31	26.7%	45	39.0%	29	25.0%	11	9.5%

Respondents reported the qualities of chaplain chart notes on a ten-point Likert scale to be: Understandable: 8.1; Substantive: 7.3; and Useful: 7.2.

Discussion

- Since no similar study of this topic could be found in the literature, these results serve as a baseline for large medical centers with solid reputations.

- About 60 percent of nurses working there either often or most of the time read a spiritual care note when they see one.

- About 45 percent of IDT respondents either *most of the time* or *often* seek available chart notes to better understand their patients, and about 55 percent *hardly ever* or *never* do.

- About 65 percent of IDT respondents either *most of the time* or *often* read a spiritual care note when they see one in the chart, while 35 percent *hardly ever* or *never* do.

- On the 1–10 scales, the average rating of IDT members regarding the quality of chaplain notes to be in the 7 and 8 range.

Conclusions and suggestions for further study

In a large hospital with chaplaincy assumed to be well integrated into units of care, this small study found that about half of the IDT members pay significant attention to what chaplains write in the charts and about 10 percent never do. Overall the study suggests that a solid percentage of clinicians are already interested in what chaplains write in the chart and it can be assumed that more would read them if spiritual care chart notes improved to better fit the mindset and daily practice patterns of healthcare clinicians' work.

The rather informal methodology used for this quality improvement study and its small sample leaves these results with little confidence of validity. A wider study using quality research procedures would need to confirm them. It can also be suggested that simply asking the survey questions promotes IDT members' interest in taking a second look at what chaplains write in the medical record.

References

Alcoholics Anonymous (1953) *Twelve Steps and Twelve Traditions. New York: Alcoholics Anonymous World Services.*

Aristotle (1869) *The Nicomachean Ethics of Aristotle. Trans. Robert Williams. London: Longmans, Green and Co.*

Berkhof, M.H., van Rijssen, J., Schellart, A.J.M., Anema, J.R., and van der Beek, A.J. (2001) "Effective training strategies for teaching communication skills to physicians: an overview of systematic reviews." *Patient Education and Counseling 84,* 152–162.

Blackmur R.P. (1983) *Studies in Henry James. New York: New Directions.*

Bolte Taylor, J. (2009) *My Stroke of Insight: A Brain Scientist's Personal Journey. New York: Plume.*

Butler, S. (1917) "Elementary Morality." In *The Note-Books of Samuel Butler. New York: E.P. Dutton & Co.*

Cassell, E.J. (2012) *The Nature of Healing: The Modern Practice of Medicine. New York: Oxford University Press.*

Charon, R. (2001) "Narrative medicine: a model for empathy, reflection, profession, and trust." *The Journal of the American Medical Association 286,* 15, 1897–1902.

Charon, R. (2008) *Narrative Medicine: Honoring the Stories of Illness. London: Oxford University Press.*

Cuddy, A. (2015) *Presence: Bringing Your Boldest Self to Your Biggest Challenges. Boston: Little, Brown and Company.*

Donne, J. (1923) *Devotions upon Emergent Occasions. Cambridge: University Press.*

Dulmus, C. and Sowers, K. (2012) *The Profession of Social Work: Guided by History, Led by Evidence.* New York: Wiley.

Egnew, T.R. (2005) "The meaning of healing: transcending suffering." *Annals of Family Medicine 3, 3,* 255–262.

Fitchett, G. and Nolan, S. (2016) *Spiritual Care in Practice: Case Studies in Healthcare Chaplaincy.* London: Jessica Kingsley Publications.

Flanelly, K., Galek, K., Handzo, G., and Jankowski, K. (2011) "A methodological analysis of chaplaincy research 2000–2009." *Journal of Health Care Chaplaincy 17,* 126–145.

Frank, A.W. (2013 [1995]) *The Wounded Storyteller: Body, Illness and Ethics.* 2nd ed. London: University of Chicago Press.

Fricchione, G. (2011) *Compassion and Healing in Medicine and Society: On the Nature and Uses of Attachment Solutions to Separation Challenges.* Baltimore: Johns Hopkins University Press.

Gawande, A. (2014) *Being Mortal: Medicine and What Matters in the End.* New York: Metropolitan Books.

Gottshall, Johathan (2013) *The Storytelling Animal: How Stories Make Us Human.* New York: Mariner Books.

Greenhalgh, T. and Hurwitz, B. (1999) "Narrative based medicine: why study narrative?" *The British Medical Journal 318,* 48, 48–50.

Hall, C.E. (1992) *Head and Heart: The Story of the Clinical Pastoral Education Movement.* Atlanta: Journal of Pastoral Care Publications.

Hamilton, L.M. (2015) *Florence Nightingale: A Life Inspired.* New York: Wyatt North.

Harlan, C. (2014) *Global Health Nursing: Narratives from the Field.* New York: Springer.

Hemenway, J. (1996) *Inside the Circle: A Historical and Practical Inquiry Concerning Process Groups in Clinical Pastoral Education.* Atlanta: Journal of Pastoral Care Publications.

Hilsman, G. (2010) "Tandem roles of written standards and personal virtue in appraising professional practice." *Reflective Practice: Formation and Supervision in Ministry 30,* 46–58.

Kahneman, D. (2011) *Thinking, Fast and Slow.* New York: Farrar, Straus and Giroux.

King, S.A. (2007) *Trust the Process: A History of Clinical Pastoral Education as Theological Education.* Lanham MD: University Press of America.

Kleinman, A. (1989) *The Illness Narratives: Suffering, Healing, and the Human Condition.* New York: Basic Books.

Kurtz, E. (2010 [1979]) *Not God: A History of Alcoholics Anonymous.* Center City, MN: Hazelden.

Leibovitz, L. (2014) *A Broken Hallelujah: Rock and Roll, Redemption, and the Life of Leonard Cohen.* New York: W.W. Norton.

Lewis, C.S. (1961) *A Grief Observed.* London: Faber and Faber.

Luks, A. (2001) *The Healing Power of Doing Good.* Bloomington IN: iUniverse.

MacGregor, B. (2013) *In Awe of Being Human: A Doctor's Stories from the Edge of Life and Death.* Greenbank WA: Abington Nowhere Press.

Mathieu, F. (2007) "Running on empty: compassion fatigue in health professionals." *Rehab & Community Care Medicine* 7, 1–6.

McCurdy, D.B. (2012) "Chaplains, confidentiality and the chart." *Chaplaincy Today, e-Journal of the Association of Professional Chaplains* 28, 2, 20–30.

McKenzie, J.L. (1965) *Dictionary of the Bible.* Milwaukee, WI: The Bruce Publishing Company.

Newberg, A. and Waldman, M.R. (2009) *How God Changes Your Brain.* New York: Ballantine Books.

Olson, S. (1946) "We need wilderness." *National Parks Magazine,* January–March.

Paquin, G.W. (2009) *Clinical Social Work: A Narrative Approach.* District of Columbia: Council on Social Work Education.

Peck, M.S. (2010) *Further along the Road Less Traveled: Sexuality & Spirituality.* New York: Simon and Schuster Audio.

Pellegrino, E.D. (1993) "The metamorphosis of medical ethics: a thirty year retrospective." *Journal of the American Medical Association* 269, 9, 1158–1162.

Pellegrino, E.D. and Thomasma, D.C. (1993) *The Virtues in Medical Practice.* London: Oxford University Press.

Puchalski, C. and Romer, A.L. (2000) "Taking a spiritual history allows clinicians to understand patients more fully." *Journal of Palliative Medicine* 3, 1, 129–137.

Rilke, R.M. (2011) *Letters to a Young Poet.* Trans. C. Louth. New York: Penguin Books.

Slavicek, G. (2012) "Interdisciplinary: a historical reflection." *International Journal of Humanities and Social Science* 2, 20 (Special Issue), 107–113.

Sullander, S. (2015) "The narrative perspective." *Reflective Practice: Formation and Supervision in Ministry* 35, 13–15.

Sullivan, L. (1896) "The tall office building artistically considered." *Lippincott's Monthly Magazine,* March, 403–408, available at https://archive.org/details/tallofficebuildi00sull, accessed on March 23, 2016.

Sullivan, W.F. (2014) *A Ministry of Presence: Chaplaincy, Spiritual Care and the Law.* Chicago: University of Chicago Press.

Tartaglia, A.F. (2015) "Reflections on the development and future of chaplaincy education." *Reflective Practice: Formation and Supervision in Ministry* 35, 116–133. Available at http://journals.sfu.ca/rpfs/index.php/rpfs/article/view/391/382, accessed on March 23, 2016.

Thomsen, R. (1975) *Bill W: The Absorbing and Deeply Moving Life Story of Bill Wilson, Co-founder of Alcoholics Anonymous.* New York: Harper and Rowe Publishers.

Index